Gender Difference in Diabetes

Gender Difference in Diabetes

Editor

Giancarlo Tonolo

MDPI • Basel • Beijing • Wuhan • Barcelona • Belgrade • Manchester • Tokyo • Cluj • Tianjin

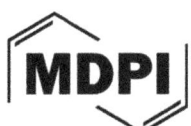

Editor
Giancarlo Tonolo
SC Diabetology ASL Gallura
Italy

Editorial Office
MDPI
St. Alban-Anlage 66
4052 Basel, Switzerland

This is a reprint of articles from the Special Issue published online in the open access journal *Diabetology* (ISSN 2673-4540) (available at: https://www.mdpi.com/journal/diabetology/special_issues/Gender_Difference_Diabetes).

For citation purposes, cite each article independently as indicated on the article page online and as indicated below:

LastName, A.A.; LastName, B.B.; LastName, C.C. Article Title. *Journal Name* **Year**, *Volume Number*, Page Range.

ISBN 978-3-0365-6790-7 (Hbk)
ISBN 978-3-0365-6791-4 (PDF)

Cover image courtesy of BIBA group srl permission

© 2023 by the authors. Articles in this book are Open Access and distributed under the Creative Commons Attribution (CC BY) license, which allows users to download, copy and build upon published articles, as long as the author and publisher are properly credited, which ensures maximum dissemination and a wider impact of our publications.

The book as a whole is distributed by MDPI under the terms and conditions of the Creative Commons license CC BY-NC-ND.

Contents

About the Editor vii

Preface to "Gender Difference in Diabetes" ix

Giancarlo Tonolo
Editorial to "Gender Differences in Diabetes"
Reprinted from: *Diabetology* 2023, 4, 62–63, doi:10.3390/diabetology4010007 1

Concetta Mezzatesta, Sara Bazzano, Rosa Gesualdo, Simone Marchese, Maria Luisa Savona, Mario Tambone Reyes and Vincenzo Provenzano
Neurocognitive Disorders in Post and Long Covid Patients: Preliminary Data, Gender Differences and New Diabetes Diagnosis
Reprinted from: *Diabetology* 2022, 3, 514–523, doi:10.3390/diabetology3040039 3

Tatiana Lai, Sofia Cincotti and Cristian Pisu
Gender Inequality and Well-Being of Healthcare Workers in Diabetology: A Pilot Study
Reprinted from: *Diabetology* 2022, 3, 384–392, doi:10.3390/diabetology3030029 13

Maria Antonietta Taras and Alessandra Pellegrini
Sex/Gender Psychological Differences in the Adult Diabetic Patient and How a Child's Response to Chronic Disease Varies with Age and Can Be Influenced by Technology
Reprinted from: *Diabetology* 2021, 2, 215–225, doi:10.3390/diabetology2040019 23

Sara Cherchi, Alfonso Gigante, Maria Anna Spanu, Pierpaolo Contini, Gisella Meloni, Maria Antonietta Fois, et al.
Sex-Gender Differences in Diabetic Retinopathy
Reprinted from: *Diabetology* 2020, 1, 1–10, doi:10.3390/diabetology1010001 35

Giuseppe Seghieri, Flavia Franconi and Ilaria Campesi
Why We Need Sex-Gender Medicine: The Striking Example of Type 2 Diabetes
Reprinted from: *Diabetology* 2022, 3, 460–469, doi:10.3390/diabetology3030034 45

Patrizio Tatti and Singh Pavandeep
Gender Difference in Type 1 Diabetes: An Underevaluated Dimension of the Disease
Reprinted from: *Diabetology* 2022, 3, 364–368, doi:10.3390/diabetology3020027 55

Federica Barbagallo, Laura M. Mongioì, Rossella Cannarella, Sandro La Vignera, Rosita A. Condorelli and Aldo E. Calogero
Sexual Dysfunction in Diabetic Women: An Update on Current Knowledge
Reprinted from: *Diabetology* 2020, 1, 11–21, doi:10.3390/diabetology1010002 61

Francesca Ena
Gender Differences in Migration
Reprinted from: *Diabetology* 2022, 3, 328–333, doi:10.3390/diabetology3020023 73

Rossella Cannarella, Federica Barbagallo, Rosita A. Condorelli, Carmelo Gusmano, Andrea Crafa, Sandro La Vignera and Aldo E. Calogero
Erectile Dysfunction in Diabetic Patients: From Etiology to Management
Reprinted from: *Diabetology* 2021, 2, 157–164, doi:10.3390/diabetology2030014 79

Giancarlo Tonolo
Sex-Gender Awareness in Diabetes
Reprinted from: *Diabetology* 2021, 2, 117–122, doi:10.3390/diabetology2020010 87

About the Editor

Giancarlo Tonolo

Tonolo Giancarlo has been the Director and Head of the Diabetology Department of ASL Gallura, Olbia, Italy, from 2008 till now, with outpatient clinics in three hospitals that serve more than 11,000 diabetic patients; his expertise is in type 1 diabetes technology (CSII, CSII-SAP, CSII-LGL, and CIIP, unique Italian center for intraperitoneal insulin infusion by DiaPort). His areas of expertise are hypertension, diabetes, and obesity in the clinical and research fields, with a particular interest in gender differences. In 2002–2003 he served as a Visiting Professor at the Medical Genetics Unit, Wallenberg Laboratory, University of Lund, Sweden. In 1984–1987 he worked as a research registrar at the MRC Blood Pressure Unit, Western Infirmary, Glasgow, UK. He has also been a Visiting Professor at the University of Harare, Zimbabwe, performing research on type 2 diabetes; he has worked at Sassari University and served as the Principal Investigator of more than 20 international RCTs by 2008. In this scientific field, he is the author or co-author of more than 200 publications in international journals, of which 131 are quoted in PubMed. He is interested in sailing. In 2018, he participated in the ARC (race from the Canaries to Martinique, with a transatlantic crossing) with a crew of eight type 1 diabetic patients, arriving sixth out of 182 participating sailing boats.

Preface to "Gender Difference in Diabetes"

Sex and gender can affect the incidence, prevalence, symptoms, course and response to drug therapy in many illnesses, with sex (the biological side) and gender (the social–cultural one) being variously interconnected. During the two days of the meeting "Gender Differences in Diabetic Disease" held in Olbia, Italy, on 4 and 5 December 2020, we discussed the various medical, social, ethnic, psychological and anthropological aspects of gender differences to build as broad a picture as possible of how these differences are present and evident in diabetic disease. Type 2 diabetes is the perfect example to justify gender medicine. During the meeting, we also tried to identify the still-unclear points that deserve further studies. As Guest Editor of this Special Issue of *Diabetology*, "The Gender Differences in Diabetic Disease", I invite you to read it. The book comes from the efforts of numerous researchers in the field and represent a small picture of what was presented at the meeting.

Giancarlo Tonolo
Editor

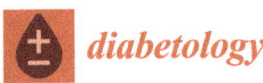

Editorial

Editorial to "Gender Differences in Diabetes"

Giancarlo Tonolo

Diabetology, San Giovanni di Dio, Via A Moro, ASL Gallura, 07026 Olbia, Italy; giancarlo.tonolo@aslgallura.it

Welcome to this Special Issue of Diabetology entitled "Gender Difference in Diabetes". Sex and gender can affect incidence, prevalence, symptoms, course, and response to drug therapy in many illnesses, considering how both sex (the biological side) and gender (the social-cultural one) are variously interconnected. In this collection of papers, you will find many articles addressing the issue of gender differences in diabetes from various perspectives. In particular, one review [1] considers and explains how type 2 diabetes is a perfect example for justifying gender medicine. Many aspects of type 2 diabetes gender differences have been uncovered, relating to pathogenesis, therapy, and complications; however, another review examines the more ambiguous and obscure aspects of gender differences in type 1 diabetes [2]: a disease already anomalous in itself for being the only form of autoimmune disease that predominantly affects young males rather than older females, distinguishing it from all other forms of autoimmunity. Another article deals with the psychological aspects of the diabetic disease from a gender perspective from the perspective of adults while also highlighting a particular, often obsolete form called diabulimia and from the perspective of the adolescent, particularly when struggling with technology [3]. Two reviews take into consideration disorders of the sexual sphere, both in men [4] and those more vastly unknown, understudied, and, therefore, less treated in women [5]. The latter takes into consideration the prevalence, etiology, diagnostic approaches, and current treatment options for female sexual dysfunction in diabetic patients. An original article explores gender differences in a common complication of diabetes, diabetic retinopathy, in an extremely large sample of 20,000 patients [6]. Last but not least, the often-marginal aspects of gender differences in migration are also explored as a function of diabetes [7]. The conclusion to this work is that health education for the population as a whole and of women specifically is needed to contain risk behavior and prevent the early onset of metabolic syndromes in general and of type 2 diabetes in migrants. Given the unprecedented times we are going through, an article reports the data of a COVID-19 unit in Italy experiencing a new onset of diabetes and the psychic damage created by the disease and how they can be connected with anatomical lesions [8]. The authors of this article raise the possibility that the presence of cognitive alterations may be related to the evidence of point-like brain alterations (from the cortex to the trunk) that are visible through neuroimaging techniques. Sex-gender differences in diabetes healthcare workers are also taken into consideration in this Special Issue: healthcare workers and how they perceive their work environment, especially in the context of the presence or absence of gender inequality [9].

In conclusion, a sex-gender approach in medicine is mandatory to maximize scientific rigor and the value of research. Sex-gender studies need interdisciplinarity and intersectionality in order to offer the most appropriate care to each person, and this Special Issue aims to contribute to this important aspect of medicine.

Enjoy the reading!

Conflicts of Interest: The author declares no conflict of interest.

Citation: Tonolo, G. Editorial to "Gender Differences in Diabetes". *Diabetology* **2023**, *4*, 62–63. https://doi.org/10.3390/diabetology4010007

Received: 28 January 2023
Accepted: 31 January 2023
Published: 3 February 2023

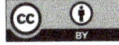

Copyright: © 2023 by the author. Licensee MDPI, Basel, Switzerland. This article is an open access article distributed under the terms and conditions of the Creative Commons Attribution (CC BY) license (https://creativecommons.org/licenses/by/4.0/).

References

1. Seghieri, G.; Franconi, F.; Campesi, I. Why We Need Sex-Gender Medicine: The Striking Example of Type 2 Diabetes. *Diabetology* **2022**, *3*, 460–469. [CrossRef]
2. Tatti, P.; Pavandeep, S. Gender Difference in Type 1 Diabetes: An Underevaluated Dimension of the Disease. *Diabetology* **2022**, *3*, 364–368. [CrossRef]
3. Taras, M.A.; Pellegrini, A. Sex/Gender Psychological Differences in the Adult Diabetic Patient and How a Child's Response to Chronic Disease Varies with Age and Can Be Influenced by Technology. *Diabetology* **2021**, *2*, 215–225. [CrossRef]
4. Barbagallo, F.; Mongioì, L.M.; Cannarella, R.; La Vignera, S.; Condorelli, R.A.; Calogero, A.E. Sexual Dysfunction in Diabetic Women: An Update on Current Knowledge. *Diabetology* **2020**, *1*, 11–21. [CrossRef]
5. Cannarella, R.; Barbagallo, F.; Condorelli, R.A.; Gusmano, C.; Crafa, A.; La Vignera, S.; Calogero, A.E. Erectile Dysfunction in Diabetic Patients: From Etiology to Management. *Diabetology* **2021**, *2*, 157–164. [CrossRef]
6. Cherchi, S.; Gigante, A.; Spanu, M.A.; Contini, P.; Meloni, G.; Fois, M.A.; Pistis, D.; Pilosu, R.M.; Lai, A.; Ruiu, S.; et al. Sex-Gender Differences in Diabetic Retinopathy. *Diabetology* **2020**, *1*, 1–10. [CrossRef]
7. Ena, F. Gender Differences in Migration. *Diabetology* **2022**, *3*, 328–333. [CrossRef]
8. Mezzatesta, C.; Bazzano, S.; Gesualdo, R.; Marchese, S.; Savona, M.L.; Reyes, M.T.; Provenzano, V. Neurocognitive Disorders in Post and Long Covid Patients: Preliminary Data, Gender Differences and New Diabetes Diagnosis. *Diabetology* **2022**, *3*, 514–523. [CrossRef]
9. Lai, T.; Cincotti, S.; Pisu, C. Gender Inequality and Well-Being of Healthcare Workers in Diabetology: A Pilot Study. *Diabetology* **2022**, *3*, 384–392. [CrossRef]

Disclaimer/Publisher's Note: The statements, opinions and data contained in all publications are solely those of the individual author(s) and contributor(s) and not of MDPI and/or the editor(s). MDPI and/or the editor(s) disclaim responsibility for any injury to people or property resulting from any ideas, methods, instructions or products referred to in the content.

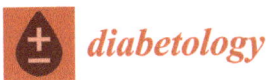

Article

Neurocognitive Disorders in Post and Long Covid Patients: Preliminary Data, Gender Differences and New Diabetes Diagnosis

Concetta Mezzatesta [1,*], Sara Bazzano [2], Rosa Gesualdo [2], Simone Marchese [1], Maria Luisa Savona [1], Mario Tambone Reyes [3] and Vincenzo Provenzano [2]

1 Psicologo Psicoterapeuta P.O. "Civico" Partinico Covid Hospital, 90047 Partinico, Italy
2 Psicologo P.O. "Civico" Partinico Covid Hospital, 90047 Partinico, Italy
3 Responsabile Long Covid Center P.O. "Civico" Partinico Covid Hospital, 90047 Partinico, Italy
* Correspondence: cettina.mezzatesta@gmail.com

Abstract: The research is based on a clinical observation of the neurological and neuro-cognitive status of 300 patients, belonging to the Partinico Hospital and the Post-Long Covid clinic, which had contracted the SARS-CoV-2 virus in the period between April 2021 and May 2022. In this paper, we present the analysis of the first 100 patients subjected to a neurocognitive screening protocol. The procedure consists of tests that examine the mechanism of different brain domains to check for the presence of cognitive deficits that arose after the negativization of the viral infection. Through a neurocognitive protocol, the research aims to investigate different brain areas and mental functioning. This allowed us to raise the possibility that the presence of cognitive alterations may be related to the evidence of point-like brain alterations (from the cortex to the trunk) visible through neuroimaging techniques. In the article, we highlight the hypothesis that SARS-covid 2, as stated in recently published studies, can produce an alteration of executive functions such as to configure a real dysexecutive syndrome. This research evaluates the symptomatic gender variability within the sample, the presence of important differences in the affective state, and provides a first observation of the impact of SARS-CoV-2 in diabetic pathology as well.

Keywords: neuroCovid; cognitive disorders; gender; Covid; long covid; diabetes; disexecutive syndrome

Citation: Mezzatesta, C.; Bazzano, S.; Gesualdo, R.; Marchese, S.; Savona, M.L.; Reyes, M.T.; Provenzano, V. Neurocognitive Disorders in Post and Long Covid Patients: Preliminary Data, Gender Differences and New Diabetes Diagnosis. *Diabetology* **2022**, *3*, 514–523. https://doi.org/10.3390/diabetology3040039

Academic Editor: Giancarlo Tonolo

Received: 4 August 2022
Accepted: 16 September 2022
Published: 6 October 2022

Publisher's Note: MDPI stays neutral with regard to jurisdictional claims in published maps and institutional affiliations.

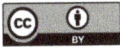

Copyright: © 2022 by the authors. Licensee MDPI, Basel, Switzerland. This article is an open access article distributed under the terms and conditions of the Creative Commons Attribution (CC BY) license (https://creativecommons.org/licenses/by/4.0/).

1. Introduction

The SARS-CoV-2 infection has revolutionized scientific paradigms, forcing healthcare professionals to return to the research-intervention model. Gradually, they had to modify their actions and adapt to events, emergencies, and new patient care criteria. The Covid patient is a complex patient with multifactorial and multidimensional symptoms requiring interventions from different branches of specialist medicine [1].

Studies in recent months showed that the psychophysical sequelae of SARS-Cov 2 infection are diversified, and often show symptoms that can be superimposed on different syndromic pictures [2–5]. As observed in recent publications, one of the long-term consequences of Covid is an alteration in cognitive functions, which can lead to multiple disorders such as memory deficits (re-enactment, fixation, and sequencing), attention deficit (immediate and sustained), a deficit in language production and understanding, decoding and execution of programming elements [6–8].

In our view, a careful neurocognitive evaluation allows highlighting the damaged mechanisms and the still-intact processes. The detection of brain regions through neuroimaging techniques (MRI, magnetic resonance imaging), might contribute to determining the relationships between neurocognitive deficits and structural/functional damage [9,10]. Starting from the study published in PLOS ONE, in February 2021 by the IRCCS San

Raffaele Hospital [11], our clinical observation allowed us to observe a further symptom picture characterized by a significant cognitive alteration linked to short and long-term memory, an alteration of attention processes, significantly impaired concentration, planning, abstraction and sensitivity to interference.

Reviewing last year's publications and clinical evidence, the research group of Psychologists and Psychotherapists of Partinico Hospital formulated a neurocognitive protocol that aims to investigate different brain areas and mental functioning.

The aim of the study is to observe three substantial elements:

- ☐ The possible presence of encephalic alterations (from the cortex to the brain stem), was verified through neuroimaging techniques, and the possible correlations with neurological alterations and neurocognition were found via the tests.
- ☐ The hypothesis is that Covid neuroinflammation, as ascertained by recently published studies, can also produce an alteration of executive functions such as to configure a real dysexecutive syndrome. In this paper, we will focus on this second point.
- ☐ Observation in the sample of the presence/absence of diabetic pathology, diabetes with the post-Covid onset, and the correlations between emerging diabetes and mood alterations (depression/anxiety), and executive functions with particular attention to gender differences.

Many studies currently support and confirm the neuro-inflammatory aspect presented by SARS-CoV-2 COVID-19 disease [12–14]. A recent study by Dr. Arianna Di Stadio [15] highlights how the histological, neuroradiological, and clinical aspects of patients affected by the virus "show that, regardless of its origin directly linked to the virus or to the systemic consequences caused by it, patients suffer from brain inflammation".

Prolonged exposure to infection, or the severity of the syndrome, may produce neurocognitive effects measurable by tests. These will be correlated both with the direct observation of executive functions (with the relative onset of cognitive deficit) and with the neuroinflammation observable through neuroimaging (MRI). Jeffrey S. Fine and his collaborators recently published a very interesting study for cognitive disorders, with a specific focus on the cognitive symptoms of PASC (post-acute sequelae of SARS-CoV-2 infection) that can occur in people diagnosed with an acute COVID19 infection. These patients (hospitalized) experienced mild to severe symptoms.

The authors of this study propose to observe in patients.

> *neurological and neuropsychiatric symptoms in individuals with PASC include fatigue, myalgia, headaches, sleep disturbance, anxiety, depression, dizziness, anosmia, dysgeusia, and cognitive symptoms, often called a brain fog. It is important for clinicians to recognize that disease severity may not be a predictor of PASC symptoms as many patients presenting to outpatient COVID recovery centers experienced only mild initial SARS-CoV-2 infection. Primary cognitive symptoms include deficits in reasoning, problem solving, spatial planning, working memory, difficulty with word retrieval, and poor attention. In addition, small studies in patients recovering from COVID-19 who develop postural orthostatic tachycardia syndrome (POTS) have shown worsening executive function and attention in the standing position.13 Assessment and treatment of cognitive symptoms in patients with PASC is the focus of this review."*

In diabetic pathology, new studies show that the COVID-19 virus can attack the pancreas by destroying insulin-producing cells and, in some cases, cause diabetes.

A meta-analysis conducted in 2020 by health researcher Thirunavukkarasu Sathish at McMaster University in Canada [16] found that nearly 15% of patients who contracted a severe form of COVID-19 also developed diabetes. However, he adds, "this number is likely higher among individuals at greater risk, for example, those with prediabetes".

The research, conducted by endocrinologist Paolo Fiorina at Harvard Medical School, and published in 2021, showed that, in a group of 551 patients hospitalized for COVID-19 in Italy, half of them developed hyperglycemia.

Peter Jackson, a biochemist at Stanford University School of Medicine, estimates that "the percentage of patients with severe COVID-19 who can develop diabetes reaches 30%".

Chen and Jackson found the connection between COVID-19 and newly onset diabetes. Both have launched independent investigations to find out how SARS-CoV-2 might trigger hyperglycemia. Both groups published their results in the May issue of the scientific journal Cell Metabolism.

Chen's group grew different types of tissue in the lab, to see which ones were vulnerable to the COVID-19 virus; surprisingly they found that the beta cells of the pancreas are very permeable to SARS-CoV-2 infection and produce higher insulin levels by altering sugar metabolism. Their findings offer an essential insight into the basic mechanisms by which COVID-19 can lead to the development of new cases of diabetes in infected patients. The group is currently working on the possibility that the hyperglycemia produced by the covid viral infection might alter the activation of HPA and be responsible for the prolongation of diabetes. If Chen's hypothesis (on a possible prolongation of diabetes linked to glycemic and HPA alteration in covid patients) were confirmed, researchers will have to evaluate the possibility that there could be a cognitive alteration linked to the hypothalamic-locus coeruleus axis.

Our research has been structured on the bases of clinical observation of the neurological and neuro-cognitive state of the covid patient during the hospitalization period.

Patients experienced brain fog, loss of attention, and both short- and long-term memory problems. In order to better understand this phenomenon, the research team structured a protocol aimed at investigating different brain areas and mental functioning. This allowed us to provide objective evidence and quantify the presence of cognitive alterations. The hypothesis of this research is that the infection of SARS CoV 2 produces alterations to executive functions (point brain alterations from the cerebral cortex to the brain stem, visible through neuroimaging techniques), alterations of the affective state and that these variations can be quantified through the neurocognitive protocol.

At the same time, the research focused on the presence, within the sample, of subjects with diabetes (also new onset diabetes), observing the characteristics of the affective state, the presence/absence of alterations in cognitive functions, and gender variations.

2. Methods

2.1. Patients

The research involves the recruitment of 300 subjects who have contracted from April 2021 to February 2022. After the communication of the research plan to the Ethics Committee of the Policlinico Hospital of Palermo, the neurocognitive protocol was administered to the sample hospitalized at the "Civico" P.O. of Partinico with an average hospital stay of 22 days (20% of them were also hospitalized in Intensive Care with an average hospital stay of 10 days) and reviewed at the Post-Long Covid Clinic in the Day Service. The analysis of the first 100 patients tested is the subject of this paper. The neurocognitive screening protocol consists of tests that examine the mechanism of different brain domains in order to check for the presence of cognitive deficits that arose after the negativization of the viral infection.

The subjects (100 patients, 63 males, and 37 females), admitted to covid hospital from April 2021 to February 2022, with an average age of 60 years, (42% diabetic) underwent psychodiagnostics interviews and were administered tested with neurocognitive tests.

2.2. Phases

The research is divided into four phases.

- The first is the administration of the first level protocol [17] with Mini Mental State Examination (MMSE), Immediate and deferred Rey figure, Frontal assessment battery (FAB), Hamilton D, Stay X and Y, Impact of Event Scale–Revised (IES). Each neuropsychological test will be corrected for gender, age, and schooling as required by international guidelines [18].

- Patients found affected by cognitive alterations moved to the second phase of the research with the administration of a second level protocol [17] with the Short Neuropsychological Exam, Davinson Trauma Scale (DTS)-800 (evaluates the 17 symptoms of PTSD) and SF-36 (a questionnaire that aims to quantify health status and measure health-related quality of life).
- The third phase is a correlation study between the test results and the finding of organic alterations in Neuroimaging [19].
- In the fourth phase, the aim is to submit people with a dysexecutive syndrome to a structured cognitive rehabilitation protocol, in association with new embodiment studies for the rehabilitation of executive functions, intervening on the damaged domains.

The expected duration is one year, making retests after 6 and 12 months to evaluate the presence of variations.

2.3. First Level Instruments

The MMSE; consisting of thirty items that are related to seven different cognitive areas: orientation in time, orientation in space, recording of words, attention and calculation, re-enactment, language, and constructional praxis. The total score goes from a minimum of 0 and a maximum of 30 points. Cut off: 25–30 points: normal cognition 21–24 points: mild dementia 10–20 points: moderate dementia 9 points or less: severe dementia.

The Figure of Rey Direct and Deferred evaluates visual spatial function, its perceptual organization and the visual memory of work and re-enactment. Cut off: Copy >28 recall > 6.2.

FAB is a first-level screening battery examining global executive functioning, composed of cognitive and behavioural evidence. It includes the conceptualization of similarities and abstraction, mental flexibility and the use of self-organizational strategies, programming, planning and organization of behaviours, sensitivity to interference, inhibitory control, and ability to manage impulsiveness and environmental autonomy. Cut off >12.

Hamilton D test (depression); it explores and evaluates depressive symptoms regardless of the psychopathological-clinical context in which it is placed. The HAM-D items are graded, some at 3 (0–2) and others at 5 (0–4) levels of severity, and each level is associated with a fairly precise and comprehensive definition. Cut off: <7 normal/absence, 8–17 mild depression, 18–24 moderate depression, <25 severe depression.

STAI: In the X and Y, form it is composed of 40 items, where 20 items measure state anxiety and the others 20 trait anxiety. State anxiety refers to an emotional state at a given time, while trait anxiety refers to a personality trait that characterizes different people. <40 normal/absence, 40–50 mild anxiety, 50–60 moderate anxiety, <60 severe anxiety.

(IES-R); evaluates the presence of post-traumatic disorders. Cut off for Avoidance 0–0.5 normal, 0.5–1.00 mild, 1.01–2.49 moderate, 2.5–4 severe; intrusion 0–0.5 normal, 0.5–1.00 mild, 1.01–2.49 moderate, 2.5–4 sever; Hyperarousal 0–0.5 normal, 0.5–1.00 mild, 1.01–2.49 moderate, 2.5–4 severe.

2.4. Second Level Instruments

ENB-2, a short neuropsychological exam (Mondini, Mapelli, Vestri, Arcara, Bisiacchi, 2011), consisting of the following tests: Digit Span, Trail Making test (TMT version A and version B), Drawing copy, interference memory (10 and 30 s), Abstraction, Token test, Prose memory (immediate and deferred), Tangled figure test, Spontaneous drawing, Phonemic fluency, Cognitive estimations, Praxis tests, Clock test, Corsi's test, Rey's wordlist, Attentional matrices. Davinson Trauma Scale DTS-800 and SF 36.

For the assessment of the presence of diabetes, 100 medical records were examined to verify: the presence/absence of diabetic pathology, the presence/absence of new onset diabetes in post-Covid (parameters: patients that after six months maintain a glycate >of 7 and basal blood glucose of 140), the characteristics of the affective state, the presence of alterations in cognitive functions, the variations between genders.

2.5. Statistical Analysis

The statistical analysis was conducted on the first results of a sample of 100 subjects (the research foresees 300 subjects in all). Descriptive statistics (mean, standard deviation (SD), minimum, median, and maximum) will be used for the continuous/quantitative variables, while frequency tables will be used for the categorical ones.

3. Results

In agreement with the international scientific data published in the last year, the results show pictures of significant cognitive alterations and different mood alterations (Figure 1).

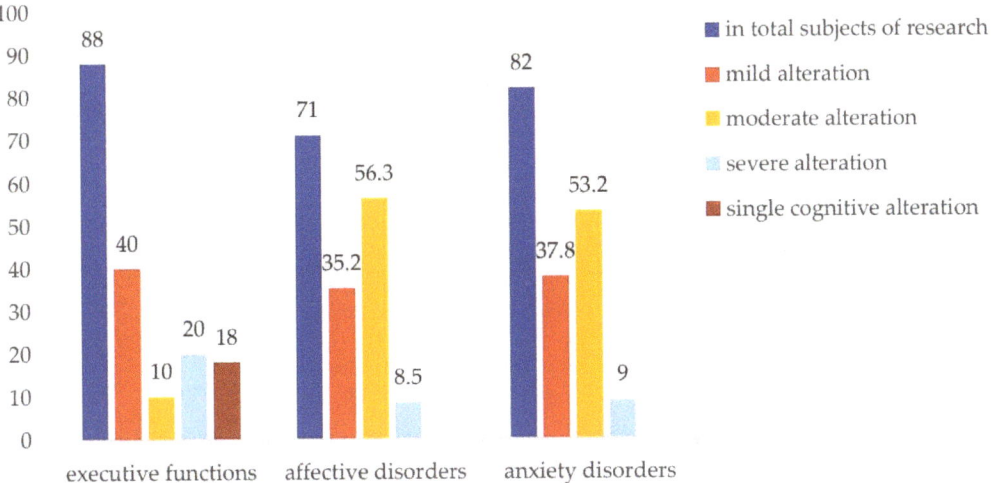

Figure 1. Mild/moderate/severe scores are percentages calculated on the total score of the individual alterations.

3.1. Cognitive Alterations

40% of the sample showed mild alterations in executive functions, with an MMSE >24 to 21 CS (correct score) correct for sex and age-CS ($\bar{x}$ 19.84, DS 1.86) Fab < 12 CS–9 CS. ($\bar{x}$ 10.6 DS 1.11) Rey Complex Figure Copy from 28 to 20 ($\bar{x}$ 23.5 DS 2.80) CS Recall from 6 to 4 CS. ($\bar{x}$ 5.09 DS 0.22).

18% showed a moderate deficit of executive functions with MMSE between 20 CS to 10 ($\bar{x}$ 17.84, DS 1.86) Fab scores between 9 and 6. ($\bar{x}$ 8.6 DS 0.22) Scores to the Figure of Rey copies from 19 to 12 CS ($\bar{x}$ 14.09 DS 1.55). Recall from <4 to 2 CS ($\bar{x}$ 3.09 DS 0.47).

10% showed a severe deficit of executive functions with MMSE between < 9 CS ($\bar{x}$ 8.47, DS 0.26) Fab <6 CS ($\bar{x}$ 5.07 DS 0.31) Rey Complex Figure Copy < 12 ($\bar{x}$ 10.5 DS 1.08) CS Recall < 2. ($\bar{x}$ 1.5 DS 0.32).

20% of the total sample showed an alteration of individual domains (attention 20%, concentration 13%, MBT and MLT 50%, sensitivity to interference 8.9%) without exceeding the cut off of MMSE and FAB, Rey. These isolated elements do not allow to make a diagnosis of dysexecutive functions. However, these clinical elements will have to be taken into account for future observation to verify that isolated alterations remain over time. 88% of the total sample had cognitive alterations.

There are no significant differences in cognitive alterations between men and women ($p > 0.05$).

3.2. Mood Disorder: Anxiety e Affective Disorders

In the evaluation of the tests that quantified the mood alterations, we verified that Mood disorders are present in 71% of the total sample; 35.2% of these are characterized by a mild depressive alteration, the remaining 56.3% by moderate depression, and 8.5% by severe depression.

An interesting fact is connected to an affective alteration of an anxious nature with STAI X Y; in fact, 82% of the sample reported clinically significant anxiety symptoms, i.e., scores greater than the cut off of <40. Within the percentage of anxious subjects, 37.8% showed mild anxiety 53.2% showed moderate anxiety, and 9% severe anxiety. Common symptoms include initial and central insomnia, irritability, psychomotor agitation and restlessness, constant state of tension, and getting scared too easily or at inappropriate times.

Gender differences: The level of significance for gender differences is high ($p < 0.01$), with higher levels of anxiety and moderate depression in women than in men; males are found to be in the mild range in both anxiety disorder and depressive disorder. The difference in the range in severe pathology is not statistically significant (Table 1).

Table 1. Gender difference in mood disorders.

	Depression Disorders					
	Mild		Moderate		Severe	
N 17	M	F	M	F	M	F
	20	5	28	25	4	2
	Anxiety Disorder					
	Mild		Moderate		Severe	
N 82	M	F	M	F	M	F
	25	4	20	29	3	1

3.3. Post Traumatic Stress Disorders

The presence of an acute posttraumatic disorder (the diagnosis is made if the symptoms persist for more than a month, and cause a significant amount of stress and difficulty in functioning) was found in 20% of the sample. In this situation of emotional stress, the psychosomatic response was very personal. Many triggers have hyper activated some subjects, activating physiological and behavioural responses when they had to deal with a very stressful context. The data about the area of "avoidance" of the IES-R of situations that reactivate the severe trauma are very high ($\bar{x}$ 3.07 DS 0.47); the area of sensation intrusion shows results high as well ($\bar{x}$ 3.27 DS 0.27); the area of Hyperarousal shows moderate results ($\bar{x}$ 2.01 DS 0.36).

The symptoms were traumatic reactivations of past bereavement, seeing images and having thoughts, nightmares, illusions, or episodes of recurring flashbacks of the traumatic event, feeling as if reliving the traumatic event, and feeling distressed when something brings back memories of the traumatic. Men and women were compared and there were no remarkable differences in the alteration of their traumatic picture.

3.4. Neurocovid and Diabetes

The data of the sample relating to diabetic patients have highlighted the complexity of all the variables investigated.

18% of the sample has a diabetic pathology (DM 1, 2), and 6% of the population has been diagnosed with new-onset diabetes. The data related to anxiety disorder in diabetics are the same as in the general sample. Data on depressive disorder must be differentiated. (Table 2).

Table 2. Mood disorders e executive functions in diabetes and in new onset diabetes.

Diabetes Subjected	Mood Disorders						Executive Functions			
	Mild		Moderate		Sever		Mild		Sever	
	M	F	M	F	M	F	M	F	M	F
Base line 12	11%	11%	22%	11%	11%	0%	11%	18%	29%	31%
New onset diabetes N 6	0%	0%	0.11%	0.06%	0.11%	0.06%	0%	0%	60%	40%

After contracting COVID 19, a higher percentage of patients previously diagnosed with diabetes, especially male patients, are more likely to present moderate depressive symptoms, with a prevalence of the male gender. The feelings predominantly experienced by the male population are connected to a perception of "uselessness" and "brachypsychism". Women experience more insomnia, "tachypsychism" and sadness. The scientific literature. [20] identifies the presence of a cognitive alteration in 23% of diabetic patients. The results of our sample show the presence of cognitive alterations in 66% (52% moderate and 14% mild alterations) of the cases observed. Even more significant is the correlation between new-onset diabetes and executive functions. Cognitive alterations are severe in 100% of patients.

4. Discussion

Cognitive functions are the set of conscious and unconscious characteristics and processes that allow human beings to identify, process, memorize, recall, use and communicate information in daily life and characterize their quality of life. Executive Functions refer to the cognitive abilities involved in initiating, planning, organizing, and regulating behaviors (Stuss & Benson, 1986). The term indicates a series of cognitive processes that interact with each other to initiate thoughts and organize functional actions to achieve a purpose (Shallice, 1994; Benso, 2010), providing the subject with the skills necessary to manage their behavior. Direct viral, secondary inflammatory, and secondary metabolic pathologies can affect this indispensable psychic functioning, altering the quality of life, and changing the relationships of patients. COVID may cause such changes through all of these three means.

There are thousands of publications about SARS-CoV 2 infection, but we are just starting to study and understand the real impact and the pathology of post and long covid [20].

This is the first study that deals with correlating executive functions (using specific broad-spectrum tests) in post and long covid subjects.

An analysis of the results of the first phase confirms the preliminary hypothesis about the presence of mild and moderate cognitive disorders in 68% of the sample, without gender differences. In post- and long-Covid patients there was a deficit of cognitive flexibility, attention and concentration deficit, working and planning memory deficit and, in some cases, problem solving deficit, deficits in judgment and decision skills, defects in empathy, deficit of interference control with difficulties of abstraction and categorization up to perseveration.

All the skills examined are attributable to the frontal and prefrontal cortex, responsible for executive functions.

The study is currently in progress but the findings in MRI of frontal gliotic foci have already been ascertained.

These first results are partly in line with what emerged from San Raffaele's research in the 2021 article in which the MRI confirmed the presence of cognitive alteration, depressive, and anxiety disorders in COVID-19 patients.

> "This is the first study that correlates functional connectivity, the structure of the white matter, the local volume of the grey matter and affective state. The rise of depressive symptoms in patients who survive the hyper-inflammatory forms of Covid-19 should not

be underestimated. It is a condition whose duration will have to be verified over time, and which could also explain the cognitive problems that usually accompany long-COVID"

As for the alteration of the affective state, the emerging data confirm the condition already expressed in November 2021 in the aforementioned study. However, the quantification emerging from our research shows a clear picture of the presence of post-Covid alterations in both the depressive type (higher percentage in women), and the anxious type (higher percentage in women). The observational study has an element of weakness: the gender variable cannot be measured. The presence of interactions was exposed in percentages.

The data referable to the presence of a high index of post-traumatic stress disorder (20% of the sample) in hospitalized tested patients, in the post and long Covid in an outpatient setting, were quite predictable.

Even if no significant differences were observed between males and females, clinicians developed a hypothesis, a result of the observation of patients over time, stating that different affective states (see results) can induce the traumatic picture to evolve in a different way. The environmental and relational variables that will intervene over time (resumption of one's own pace of work, resilience, and family environment) will be decisive for the prolongation of the post-traumatic disorder.

Two observations about data on diabetes. The first concerns the presence of a new post-Covid diabetic pathology as an element that provides for further research and in-depth analysis [18,21–31]. The second observation is related to the comorbidity of depression and cognitive functions. Right now, the long-term effects of covid are the real clinical challenge of the coming years. First observation: Data that emerged shows that patients with new onset diabetes are complex patients also from a neurocovid point of view (Table 2).

The data show, in fact, that all the samples diagnosed with newly onset diabetes has a severe or moderate alteration of the mood (Tables 1 and 2), and all the newly diagnosed manifest an alteration of the executive functions (moderate and severe degree). One of the strengths of the observational study was the chance to follow patients from the moment of admission to the outpatient setting, verifying the progressive loss of some cognitive skills, then confirmed by the testological evaluation.

A further strength of our study and its continuation is the compilation of variables on cognitive function, mood disorders, and diabetes that have been investigated too little in COVID patients. The weaknesses are related to the inability to standardize the sample (and guarantee the same percentage of males' and females' samples) and the smallness of the preliminary sample.

5. Conclusions

The results of our research are comparable to the earlier data in the literature. The results of neuropsychological tests represent an evolution, a chance to quantify the cognitive states observed in clinical practice, and the neuropathological states currently studied. All the data currently collected converge towards confirmation of the hypothesis formulated by the research group regarding the presence of a post-Covid dysexecutive syndrome. This neuropsychological protocol, in association with clinical scales, represents a first evaluation that provides objective evidence and quantifies the data collected during the observation of post and long Covid patients. However, our study shows that much of the pathophysiology relating to the prolongation of covid pathology may relate not just to autoimmunity and pulmonary phenomena (as stated in recent international literature), but also to significant metabolic and neuropsychopathological alterations.

Author Contributions: Conceptualization, C.M. and M.T.R.; methodology, C.M.; software, SPSS statistics; formal analysis, all authors; investigation, S.B., R.G., S.M. and M.L.S.; writing—original draft preparation and writing—review and editing, project administration, C.M., supervision, V.P. All authors have read and agreed to the published version of the manuscript.

Funding: This research received no external funding.

Institutional Review Board Statement: Policlinico Paolo Giaccone Palermo May 2022.

Informed Consent Statement: Not applicable.

Data Availability Statement: The data presented in this study are available on request from the corresponding author.

Conflicts of Interest: The authors declare no conflict of interest.

References

1. The Lancet Neurology. The neurological impact of COVID-19. *Lancet Neurol.* **2020**, *19*, 471. [CrossRef]
2. Herman, C.; Mayer, K.; Sarwal, A. Scoping review of prevalence of neurologic comorbidities in patients hospitalized for COVID-19. *Neurology* **2020**, *95*, 77–84. [CrossRef] [PubMed]
3. Mao, L.; Jin, H.; Wang, M.; Hu, Y.; Chen, S.; He, Q.; Chang, J.; Hong, C.; Zhou, Y.; Wang, D.; et al. Neurologic manifestations of hospitalized patients with coronavirus disease 2019 in Wuhan, China. *JAMA Neurol.* **2020**, *77*, 683–690. [CrossRef]
4. Pleasure, S.J.; Green, A.J.; Josephson, S.A. The spectrum of neurologic disease in the severe acute respiratory syndrome coronavirus 2 pandemic infection: Neurologists move to the frontlines. *JAMA Neurol.* **2020**, *77*, 679–680. [CrossRef]
5. Beyrouti, R.; Adams, M.E.; Benjamin, L.; Cohen, H.; Farmer, S.F.; Goh, Y.Y.; Humphries, F.; Jäger, H.R.; Losseff, N.A.; Perry, R.J.; et al. Characteristics of ischaemic stroke associated with COVID-19. *J. Neurol. Neurosurg. Psychiatry* **2020**, *91*, 889–891. [CrossRef] [PubMed]
6. Xiong, W.; Mu, J.; Guo, J.; Lu, L.; Liu, D.; Luo, J.; Li, N.; Liu, J.; Yang, D.; Gao, H.; et al. New onset neurologic events in people with COVID-19 in 3 regions in China. *Neurology* **2020**, *95*, e1479–e1487. [CrossRef]
7. Zanin, L.; Saraceno, G.; Panciani, P.P.; Renisi, G.; Signorini, L.; Migliorati, K.; Fontanella, M.M. SARS-CoV-2 can induce brain and spine demyelinating lesions. *Acta Neurochir.* **2020**, *162*, 1491–1494. [CrossRef]
8. Zubair, A.S.; McAlpine, L.S.; Gardin, T.; Farhadian, S.; Kuruvilla, D.E.; Spudich, S. Neuropathogenesis and neurologic manifestations of the coronaviruses in the age of coronavirus disease 2019: A review. *JAMA Neurol.* **2020**, *77*, 1018–1027. [CrossRef]
9. Varatharaj, A.; Thomas, N.; Ellul, M.A.; Davies, N.W.S.; Pollak, T.A.; Tenorio, E.L.; Michael, B.D. CoroNerve Study Group. Neurological and neuropsychiatric complications of COVID-19 in 153 patients: A UK-wide surveillance study. *Lancet Psychiatry* **2020**, *7*, 875–882. [CrossRef]
10. Benussi, A.; Pilotto, A.; Premi, E.; Libri, I.; Giunta, M.; Agosti, C.; Alberici, A.; Baldelli, E.; Benini, M.; Bonacina, S.; et al. Clinical characteristics and outcomes of inpatients with neurologic disease and COVID-19 in Brescia, Lombardy, Italy. *Neurology* **2020**, *95*, e910–e920. [CrossRef] [PubMed]
11. Alemanno, F.; Houdayer, E.; Parma, A.; Spina, A.; Del Forno, A.; Scatolini, A.; Angelone, S.; Brugliera, L.; Tettamanti, A.; Beretta, L.; et al. COVID-19 cognitive deficits after respiratory assistance in the subacute phase: A COVID-rehabilitation unit experience. *PLoS ONE* **2021**, *16*, e0246590. [CrossRef]
12. Beghi, E.; Helbok, R.; Crean, M.; Chou, S.H.; McNett, M.; Moro, E.; Bassetti, C.; Jenkins, T.; Oertzen, T.; Bodini, B.; et al. EAN Neuro-COVID Task Force. The European Academy of Neurology COVID-19 registry (ENERGY): An international instrument for surveillance of neurological complications in patients with COVID-19. *Eur. J. Neurol.* **2020**, *28*, 3303–3323. [CrossRef]
13. Helms, J.; Kremer, S.; Merdji, H.; Schenck, M.; Severac, F.; Clere-Jehl, R.; Meziani, F. Delirium and encephalopathy in severe COVID-19: A cohort analysis of ICU patients. *Crit. Care* **2020**, *24*, 491. [CrossRef] [PubMed]
14. Zádori, N.; Váncsa, S.; Farkas, N.; Hegyi, P.; Erőss, B.; KETLAK Study Group. The negative impact of comorbidities on the disease course of COVID-19. *Intensive Care Med.* **2020**, *46*, 1784–1786. [CrossRef]
15. Di Stadio, A.; Brenner, M.J.; De Luca, P.; Albanese, M.; D'Ascanio, L.; Ralli, M.; Roccamatisi, D.; Cingolani, C.; Vitelli, F.; Camaioni, A.; et al. Olfactory Dysfunction, Headache, and Mental Clouding in Adults with Long-COVID-19: What Is the Link between Cognition and Olfaction? A Cross-Sectional Study. *Brain Sci.* **2022**, *12*, 154. [CrossRef]
16. Sathish, T.; Kapoor, N.; Cao, Y.; Tapp, R.J.; Zimmet, P. Proportion of newly diagnosed diabetes in COVID-19 patients: A systematic review and meta-analysis. *Diabetes Obes. Metab.* **2021**, *23*, 870–874. [CrossRef]
17. Kandel, E.R.; Schwartz, J.H.; Jessell, T.M.; Siegelbaum, S.A.; Hudspeth, A.J.; Perri, V.; Spidalieri, G. *Principi di Neuroscienze*; Casa Editrice Ambrosiana: Milano, Italy, 2014.
18. Song, I.U.; Choi, E.K.; Oh, J.K.; Chung, Y.A.; Chung, S.W. Alteration patterns of brain glucose metabolism: Comparisons of healthy controls, subjective memory impairment and mild cognitive impairment. *Acta Radiol.* **2016**, *57*, 90–97. [CrossRef] [PubMed]
19. Joseph, S. Psychometric Evaluation of Horowitz's Impact of Event Scale: A Review. *J. Trauma Stress* **2000**, *13*, 101–113. [CrossRef]
20. Yong, S.J. Long COVID or post-COVID-19 syndrome: Putative pathophysiology, risk factors, and treatments. *Infect. Dis.* **2021**, *53*, 737–754. [CrossRef]
21. Burgmer, M.; Rehbein, M.A.; Wrenger, M.; Kandil, J.; Heuft, G.; Steinberg, C.; Junghöfer, M. Early Affective Processing in Patients with Acute Posttraumatic Stress Disorder: Magnetoencephalographic Correlates. *PLoS ONE* **2013**, *8*, e71289. [CrossRef] [PubMed]
22. Fine, J.S.; Ambrose, A.F.; Didehbani, N.; Fleming, T.K.; Glashan, L.; Longo, M.; Merlino, A.; Ng, R.; Nora, G.J.; Rolin, S.; et al. Multi-disciplinary collaborative consensus guidance statement on the assessment and treatment of cognitive symptoms in patients with post-acute sequelae of SARS-CoV-2 infection (PASC). *PM&R* **2022**, *14*, 96–111. [CrossRef]

23. Solerte, S.B.; D'Addio, F.; Trevisan, R.; Lovati, E.; Rossi, A.; Pastore, I.; Dell'Acqua, M.; Ippolito, E.; Scaranna, C.; Bellante, R.; et al. Sitagliptin Treatment at the Time of Hospitalization Was Associated With Reduced Mortality in Patients with Type 2 Diabetes and COVID-19: A Multicenter, Case-Control, Retrospective, Observational Study. *Diabetes Care* **2020**, *43*, 2999–3006. [CrossRef] [PubMed]
24. Wu, C.-T.; Lidsky, P.V.; Xiao, Y.; Lee, I.T.; Cheng, R.; Nakayama, T.; Jiang, S.; Demeter, J.; Bevacqua, R.J.; Chang, C.A.; et al. SARS-CoV-2 infects human pancreatic β cells and elicits β cell impairment. *Cell Metab.* **2021**, *33*, 1565–1576.e5. [CrossRef] [PubMed]
25. Denes, G. *Manuale di Neuropsicologia. Normalità e Patologia dei Processi Cognitivi*; Zanichelli: Bologna, Italy, 2019.
26. Ceriello, A. Hyperglycemia and COVID-19: What was known and what is really new? *Diabetes Res. Clin. Pract.* **2020**, *167*, 108383. [CrossRef]
27. Nassar, M.; Nso, N.; Gonzalez, C.; Lakhdar, S.; Alshamam, M.; Elshafey, M.; Rizzo, V. COVID-19 vaccine-induced myocarditis case report with literature review. *Diabetes Metab. Syndr. Clin. Res. Rev.* **2021**, *15*, 102205. [CrossRef]
28. Steenblock, C.; Schwarz, P.E.H.; Perakakis, N.; Brajshori, N.; Beqiri, P.; Bornstein, S.R. The interface of COVID-19, diabetes, and depression. *Discov. Ment. Health* **2022**, *2*, 5. [CrossRef]
29. Chen, J.; Wu, C.; Wang, X.; Yu, J.; Sun, Z. The impact of COVID-19 on blood glucose: A systematic review and meta-analysis. *Front. Endocrinol.* **2020**, *11*, 574541. [CrossRef]
30. Zhu, L.; She, Z.-G.; Cheng, X.; Qin, J.-J.; Zhang, X.-J.; Cai, J.; Lei, F.; Wang, H.; Xie, J.; Wang, W.; et al. Association of blood glucose control and outcomes in patients with COVID-19 and pre-existing type 2 diabetes. *Cell Metab.* **2020**, *31*, 1068–1077.e3. [CrossRef]
31. Kochhann, R.; Varela, J.S.; Lisboa, C.S.M.; Chaves, M.L.F. The Mini Mental State Examination: Review of cutoff points adjusted for schooling in a large Southern Brazilian sample. *Dement. Neuropsychol.* **2010**, *4*, 35–41. [CrossRef]

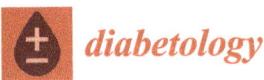

Article

Gender Inequality and Well-Being of Healthcare Workers in Diabetology: A Pilot Study

Tatiana Lai [1,*], Sofia Cincotti [2] and Cristian Pisu [3]

1. Diabetology Service, San Marcellino Hospital, 09043 Muravera, Italy
2. Independent Researcher, 09045 Quartu Sant'Elena, Italy; sofia.cincotti@tiscali.it
3. Independent Researcher, 09043 Muravera, Italy; cristian.pisu90@tiscali.it
* Correspondence: tatiana.lai73@gmail.com

Abstract: Several factors affect the relationship between a diabetic patient and a healthcare worker. Among these, there is the well-being of healthcare workers and how they perceive their work environment, especially in the context of the presence or absence of gender inequality. To show the importance of these aspects, a selected sample of healthcare workers who were exposed daily to people (mainly diabetic patients) within the working environment were interviewed. The different opinions of the interviewees show that in an environment where factors that negatively affected their work and personal well-being were minimized, healthcare workers were able to fully express their potential. They expressed great satisfaction with their work involving daily contact with patients, while achieving the type of patient–healthcare worker relationship model desired for a better management of diabetic patients' care.

Keywords: diabetology; gender inequality; healthcare worker; diabetic patient

Citation: Lai, T.; Cincotti, S.; Pisu, C. Gender Inequality and Well-Being of Healthcare Workers in Diabetology: A Pilot Study. *Diabetology* **2022**, *3*, 384–392. https://doi.org/10.3390/diabetology3030029

Academic Editor: Giancarlo Tonolo

Received: 25 March 2022
Accepted: 18 June 2022
Published: 21 June 2022

Publisher's Note: MDPI stays neutral with regard to jurisdictional claims in published maps and institutional affiliations.

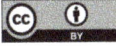

Copyright: © 2022 by the authors. Licensee MDPI, Basel, Switzerland. This article is an open access article distributed under the terms and conditions of the Creative Commons Attribution (CC BY) license (https://creativecommons.org/licenses/by/4.0/).

1. Introduction

Currently, the debate on gender inequality and healthcare workers' well-being is central. Healthcare workers are entrusted with teaching patients [1] about their diabetes and showing them how to live autonomously with the disease. The outcome of this attitude is a significant improvement in the treatment process [2]. As reported within the DAWN study [3], effective communication between the patient and the sanitary team and the subsequent improved relationship offer the prerequisite to the correct approach to overcome the comprehension and self-treatment barriers generated by the disease, and to improve the healthcare in general [4]. The synergistic work of the whole sanitary team to implement a correct coordination and collaboration attitude is the major factor in achieving this goal. The availability of an interdisciplinary team, solely established and coordinated for the diabetes treatment, has been identified as a major factor to the disease treatment [5]. Healthcare workers who interface with diabetic patients must be able to express their full potential in a healthy work environment not characterized by gender inequalities, which ultimately affect personal well-being and motivation. Listening to and understanding those healthcare workers who work primarily in contact with diabetes patients leads to an understanding of the influence of the working wellness, the gender inequality, and subsequent impact on the relationship with patients.

2. Gender Inequality in the World and in the Health Sector

According to the definition provided by the European Institute for Gender Equality, gender inequality is framed in a social and cultural state in which sex and/or gender determine different rights and dignity for men and women; this is reflected in their unequal assumption of social and cultural roles [6]. It's important to analyze the phenomenon of gender inequality from a statistical point of view in order to have a true perception of the gap in Europe and the world. The Global Gender Gap Index, elaborated in the

Global Gender Gap Report 2021, tracks the progress of gender gaps over time (it measures scores on a scale from 0 to 100 and represents the distance from parity, i.e., the percentage of the gender gap that has been bridged); in 2021, it was equal to 67.7% (calculated on 153 countries). Compared with the previous year, the gender gap widened by an average of about 0.6 percentage points. In the global ranking, Iceland and Finland showed better results in terms of gender equality: they bridged at least 85% of their gap. In general, Western Europe had the best performance, further improving its gender gap in 2021 (from 76.7% in 2020 to 77.6% in 2021) [7]. Within the European Union, women earn on average 16% less than men; this happens as women concentrate on lower-level and lower-paid jobs and are more likely to choose a part-time job. The gender pay gap among healthcare workers is particularly wide when compared with other sectors, reaching up to 33% [8]. Healthcare is one of the main global sectors comprised of women. Despite women making up about 70% of the global healthcare workforce, they are largely relegated to lower-paid sectors and jobs, with men holding most of prestigious positions. Women hold only a minority of leadership positions in the healthcare sector (25%) [9]. Addressing the issue of gender equality within healthcare workforce is important because the present disparity contributes to largely inexplicable gender pay gaps. Prejudices and discrimination constitute additional obstacles for women in the healthcare workforce, keeping them away from leadership positions by excluding them from reaching their full potential. This feeds the vicious cycle of inequality and discrimination that is already present and undermines the well-being of healthcare workers.

3. The Well-Being of Healthcare Workers in Diabetology and their Relationships with Patients

Chronic illnesses, such as diabetes, are one of the greatest health issues which must be perceived differently from a nursing point of view. Healthcare workers have a fundamental role to educate and guide patients to autonomy, which consists of learning to self-manage the disease to be able to function in a normal daily life. The new role of the diabetology team is to be an educator of patients, who have the right to be guided by a trained operator throughout their treatment. This role goes beyond purely assisting to becoming an educational guide, passing from a set of pure and simple technical notions to a real interpersonal and interdisciplinary relationship aimed at the patients' acquisition of knowledge, competence, and autonomy [10]. Therefore, education undertakes a significant role, because through education, the patient can become aware and responsible for the choices they make in maintaining a state of well-being [11].

In this contemporary era, people possess a higher cultural level. When someone turns to healthcare services, they ask to no longer undergo the dehumanizing process in which the experience of suffering and illness is simply reduced to a technical identification of a given biochemical or diseased organ. Patients are less likely to accept and undergo a health intervention in which they as a human being are not contemplated. This becomes a necessity in diabetology: the chronic patient needs to be accompanied in their treatment by a healthcare worker who exercises a relationship no longer characterized only by technical and pharmacological activities, but also by complementary non-pharmacological interventions of humanization of care that can respond to the new needs of today's patients. The center of care must be the patient, who should always feel supported, understood, and stimulated, in order to avoid conflicting and destabilizing behaviors. A "person-centered" care is essential to achieving optimal results in the treatment of diabetes [12].

Healthcare workers must improve the ability to enter into a relationship with patients (improve active listening, communication, and reception) and to identify and manage the emotional aspects; only in this way will they be able to "take care" of diabetic patients [13]. In this perspective, the work of the diabetology team is fundamental; that is, it is not limited to a pure exchange of information but is divided into a communicative process that stimulates the ability to interpret and participate with the aim of arriving at the formulation of effective strategies [14]. A cohesive diabetological team, whose objective is to achieve the best patient–healthcare worker relationship, requires the presence of a working environment in which healthcare workers are able to recognize and express their full potential. This allows them to become highly motivated and fully grasp the meaning of their work and the benefits it has on their relationships with those who need constant care and support.

4. Materials and Research Methods

To understand how gender inequality and work well-being affect the patient–healthcare worker relationship, a survey was taken on a small sample of healthcare workers who were in constant contact with diabetic patients. Chronic diabetic patients require a different approach to the treatment process that takes place in close connection with healthcare workers. The relationship between patients and healthcare workers can be influenced by the emotional approach to work assumed by the healthcare workers. The survey aimed to investigate the way healthcare workers approach this relationship and their work by exploring three related aspects: the way they perceive the phenomenon of gender inequality and how this affects their daily activities; their state of well-being; and finally their emotional approach to work (focusing on direct contact with the patient). The anonymous questionnaire was divided into four specific areas:

1. Social–personal characteristics, 6 questions;
2. Gender inequality in the work environment, 10 questions;
3. Current state of well-being, 9 questions;
4. Emotional approach to work, 14 questions.

The social–personal characteristics section aimed to understand the distribution of the personal and social characteristics of the sample, such as gender, age group (respondents were asked to choose the age group they belonged to, from 20 to 60+), educational qualifications, and the geographical area in which they worked. The gender inequality section aimed to understand the degree of agreement/disagreement of the respondent with some statements related to the presence of gender inequality in their working environment. Possible answers were formulated according to the method of the Likert scale (completely disagree, in disagreement, partially in disagreement, neither in agreement nor in disagreement, partially in agreement, in agreement, or completely in agreement) and evaluated according to the most frequent answer. Questions were not formulated to establish which gender was disadvantaged in their work environment but to understand how healthcare workers perceive and relate to the phenomenon gender inequality. The third section (current state of well-being) had the specific intent to investigate the state of well-being of the interviewee within the last month (a limited period of time to which respondents can refer to evaluate their feelings). The last section (emotional approach to work) aimed to understand the state of the well-being of healthcare workers in the context of their work through multiple-choice questions. Finally, a space dedicated to further comments (optional) for the interviewee on the gender inequality theme was included, in which it was possible to express in one sentence the personal reflection on the theme covered in the interview. The answers were analyzed through data analysis and visualization tools in order to be summarized in the corresponding sections and obtain useful information to investigate the main topic.

5. Results Obtained

The questionnaire was submitted to 176 healthcare workers who came from 34 different Italian provinces. The last optional section was filled in by about 36% of respond-ents.

5.1. Social–Personal Characteristics

As shown in Table 1, the average respondent identified as a woman between the ages of 51 and 60.

Table 1. Distribution of age range and sex.

Age Range	Women (Total and %)	Men (Total and %)	Total and %
20–35	26 (14.77%)	8 (4.54%)	34 (19.31%)
36–50	44 (25%)	12 (6.81%)	56 (31.81%)
51–60	58 (32.95%)	14 (7.95%)	72 (40.9%)
60+	10 (5.68%)	4 (2.27%)	14 (7.95%)
Total	138 (78.41%)	38 (21.59%)	176 (100%)

5.2. Gender Inequality in the Work Environment

The first question ("In the healthcare company where I work there is the phenomenon of gender inequality") directly addressed the phenomenon of gender inequality; from the answers (Table 2), it can be noted that there was no polarization of opinions between agreement or disagreement, as 50% of respondents declared that they did not perceive the phenomenon, compared with 32.38% who agreed with the statement (the remaining part remained neutral). Almost all male respondents did not perceive the phenomenon of gender inequality, while female respondents were almost equally distributed between agreed, disagreement, and impartial answers.

Table 2. In the healthcare company where I work there is the phenomenon of gender inequality.

Answers	Women (Total and %)	Men (Total and %)	Total and %
Completely disagree	16 (9.09%)	14 (7.95%)	30 (17.04%)
Disagree	28 (15.90%)	9 (5.11%)	37 (21.02%)
Partially disagree	16 (9.09%)	5 (2.84%)	21 (11.93%)
Neither in agreement nor in disagreement	26 (14.77%)	5 (2.84%)	31 (17.61%)
Partially in agreement	27 (15.34%)	2 (1.14%)	29 (16.47%)
In agreement	20 (11.36%)	2 (1.14%)	22 (12.5%)
Completely agree	5 (2.84%)	1 (0.57%)	6 (3.4%)
Total	138 (78.41%)	38 (21.59%)	176 (100%)

In the following questions, respondents took different positions regarding the presence of gender inequalities in career advancement, pay, and leadership positions. In particular, as can be seen from Table 3, the majority of respondents did not believe that men receive a higher salary than women for the same position in their company (men and women both disagreed with the statement). The percentage of respondents who did not feel either in agreement or disagreement with the statement remained high.

Table 3. In the company where I work, men receive a higher salary than women (for the same position).

Answers	Women (Total and %)	Men (Total and %)	Total and %
Completely disagree	31 (17.61%)	19 (10.79%)	50 (28.4%)
Disagree	48 (27.27%)	11 (6.25%)	59 (33.52%)
Partially disagree	7 (3.97%)	3 (1.70%)	10 (5.67%)
Neither in agreement nor in disagreement	28 (15.90%)	4 (2.27%)	32 (18.17%)
Partially in agreement	12 (6.81%)	1 (0.57%)	13 (7.38%)
In agreement	10 (5.68%)	0	10 (5.68%)
Completely agree	2 (1.14%)	0	2 (1.14%)
Total	138 (78.41%)	38 (21.59%)	176 (100%)

Respondents did not perceive that it is easier and faster for men to advance their careers to more prestigious and top positions; men disagreed with these statements, while women had different opinions (Tables 4 and 5). However, most of the respondents found that top or managerial positions are held more by men than by women (Table 6). This could confirm the claim that, in the healthcare workforce, women shun leadership positions, which prevents them from reaching their full potential. Respondents (both women and men) disagree that male candidates are preferred over female candidates for the purposes of recruitment with equal curriculum (Table 7).

Table 4. In the healthcare company where I work, career advancement is faster for men than what happens in the case of women.

Answers	Women (Total and %)	Men (Total and %)	Total and %
Completely disagree	12 (6.81%)	11 (6.25%)	23 (13.06%)
Disagree	30 (17.04%)	8 (4.54%)	38 (21.59%)
Partially disagree	13 (7.39%)	8 (4.54%)	21 (11.93%)
Neither in agreement nor in disagreement	23 (13.06%)	6 (3.41%)	29 (16.48%)
Partially in agreement	27 (15.34%)	3 (1.70%)	30 (17.04%)
In agreement	30 (17.04%)	1 (0.57%)	31 (17.61%)
Completely agree	3 (1.70%)	1 (0.57%)	4 (2.27%)
Total	138 (78.41%)	38 (21.59%)	176 (100%)

Table 5. In the healthcare company where I work, the most prestigious and important tasks are assigned more often to men than to women.

Answers	Women (Total and %)	Men (Total and %)	Total and %
Completely disagree	14 (7.95%)	10 (5.68%)	24 (13.63%)
Disagree	35 (19.88%)	13 (7.39%)	48 (27.27%)
Partially disagree	14 (7.95%)	6 (3.41%)	20 (11.36%)
Neither in agreement nor in disagreement	25 (14.20%)	4 (2.27%)	29 (16.48%)
Partially in agreement	22 (12.50%)	3 (1.70%)	25 (14.2%)
In agreement	23 (13.06%)	1 (0.57%)	24 (13.64%)
Completely agree	5 (2.84%)	1 (0.57%)	6 (3.41%)
Total	138 (78.41%)	38 (21.59%)	176 (100%)

Table 6. In the healthcare company where I work, top or management positions are held more by men than by women.

Answers	Women (Total and %)	Men (Total and %)	Total and %
Completely disagree	11 (6.25%)	7 (3.98%)	18 (10.23%)
Disagree	21 (11.93%)	8 (4.54%)	29 (16.48%)
Partially disagree	13 (7.39%)	7 (3.98%)	20 (11.36%)
Neither in agreement nor in disagreement	20 (11.36%)	7 (3.98%)	27 (15.34%)
Partially in agreement	29 (16.48%)	3 (1.70%)	32 (18.18%)
In agreement	28 (15.91%)	4 (2.27%)	32 (18.18%)
Completely agree	16 (9.09%)	2 (1.14%)	18 (10.23%)
Total	138 (78.41%)	38 (21.59%)	176 (100%)

Table 7. In the healthcare company where I work, male candidates (with the same qualifications and resumes) are preferred for the purpose of recruitment.

Answers	Women (Total and %)	Men (Total and %)	Total and %
Completely disagree	18 (10.23%)	17 (9.66%)	35 (19.89%)
Disagree	48 (27.27%)	7 (3.98%)	55 (31.25%)
Partially disagree	11 (6.25%)	3 (1.70%)	14 (7.95%)
Neither in agreement nor in disagreement	33 (18.75%)	7 (3.98%)	40 (22.73%)
Partially in agreement	12 (6.82%)	4 (2.27%)	16 (9.09%)
In agreement	14 (7.95%)	0	14 (7.95%)
Completely agree	2 (1.14%)	0	2 (1.14%)
Total	138 (78.41%)	38 (21.59%)	176 (100%)

In general, the majority of respondents (both women and men) completely disagreed with the claim that the presence of gender inequality in the workplace affects their emotional state and daily tasks (Tables 8 and 9). It is useful to report that the data show that the percentage of respondents who feel in agreement with the previous statements are placed on different age groups from 20 to 60+: the negative influence of the presence of gender inequality has no age.

Table 8. The presence of gender inequality in my healthcare company negatively affects my motivation in the workplace.

Answers	Women (Total and %)	Men (Total and %)	Total and %
Completely disagree	45 (25.57%)	18 (10.23%)	63 (35.79%)
Disagree	39 (22.16%)	7 (3.98%)	46 (26.14%)
Partially disagree	9 (5.11%)	2 (1.14%)	11 (6.25%)
Neither in agreement nor in disagreement	14 (7.95%)	4 (2.27%)	18 (10.21%)
Partially in agreement	13 (7.39%)	5 (2.84%)	18 (10.21%)
In agreement	16 (9.09%)	1 (0.57%)	17 (9.66%)
Completely agree	2 (1.14%)	1 (0.57%)	3 (1.7%)
Total	138 (78.41%)	38 (21.59%)	176 (100%)

Table 9. The presence of gender inequality in my healthcare company causes me anxiety and tension.

Answers	Women (Total and %)	Men (Total and %)	Total and %
Completely disagree	43 (24.43%)	16 (9.09%)	59 (33.52%)
Disagree	36 (20.45%)	9 (5.11%)	45 (25.57%)
Partially disagree	12 (6.82%)	5 (2.84%)	17 (9.66%)
Neither in agreement nor in disagreement	17 (9.66%)	5 (2.84%)	22 (12.5%)
Partially in agreement	18 (10.22%)	1 (0.57%)	19 (10.79%)
In agreement	9 (5.11%)	1 (0.57%)	10 (5.68%)
Completely agree	3 (1.70%)	1 (0.57%)	4 (2.27%)
Total	138 (78.41%)	38 (21.59%)	176 (100%)

5.3. State of Current Well-Being

The interviewees' state of well-being was characterized, for about 29%, by a state of anxiety and nervousness that does not affect daily tasks. On the other hand, the remaining part did not perceive a state of anxiety and nervousness or perceived in only slightly (Table 10). The state of anxiety and worry varied among respondents: 42% said they had never been in such a state in the last month, 27.8% said they felt anxiety and worry half the time, and up to 17% found themselves in a state of anxiety most of the time. Just under half of the respondents said they had never felt down in the last month and that they had been mostly cheerful and felt motivated and confident most of the time. However, it is worth noting that among respondents, 13.1% felt a lack of energy, and 12.5% felt down most of the time. Similar percentages were obtained for the states of lacking joy, motivation, and self-confidence. Although most interviewees demonstrated a high state of personal well-being, there remained a small number of healthcare workers who experienced states of anxiety, worry, low motivation, and self-confidence.

Respondents who declared that (in the last month) they had almost never found themselves in a state of anxiety and worry and that they felt motivated and self-confident did not particularly perceive the phenomenon of gender inequality in their company.

Table 10. In the last month have you ever felt a state of tension and nervousness?

Answers	Total and %
Absolutely yes, not to be able to take care of my daily tasks	14 (7.95%)
Yes, but it did not affect my daily tasks	51 (28.98%)
Enough	47 (26.7%)
Slightly	34 (19.32%)
By no means	30 (17.04%)
Total	176 (100%)

5.4. Emotional Approach to Work

In general, for the most healthcare workers, interfacing with patients was simple and effective: 54.54% of respondents said they easily understood what their patients thought often during the week, and 26.14% said they could always understand their patients (Table 11). Almost all respondents managed to effectively address their patients' problems during the week by making them feel comfortable (Tables 12 and 13). From the answers analyzed, we found that the healthcare workers understood the importance of their role in front of patients and the value that this can bring in the path of care. In fact, interviewees thought they had accomplished useful things through their work either almost always (63.64%) or always (32.95%) (Table 14). Working in contact with people was a source of satisfaction every day of the week for 46% of the interviewees and often during the week for 32.38% (Table 15). However, a significant proportion of respondents said they often felt fatigued during the week (35.2% often during the week, and 15.3% every day of the week). Working in contact with people did not appear to be tiring for most of the interviewees (Table 16).

The comments on the optional section highlighted that, although the issue of gender inequality was considered important by the healthcare workers, they considered their workplace (in particular, diabetology) a place where they could express their potential as people and as professionals.

Table 11. I easily understand how my users think.

Answers	Total and %
Never	4 (2.27%)
Rarely during the week	8 (4.54%)
Half the time during the week	9 (5.11%)
Occasionally during the week	13 (7.39%)
Often throughout the week	96 (54.54%)
Every day of the week	46 (26.14%)
Total	176 (100%)

Table 12. I can effectively deal with my users' problems.

Answers	Total and %
Never	1 (0.57%)
Rarely during the week	1 (0.57%)
Half the time during the week	6 (3.41%)
Occasionally during the week	11 (6.25%)
Often throughout the week	103 (58.52%)
Every day of the week	54 (30.68%)
Total	176 (100%)

Table 13. With my way of posing I think I can make my users feel at ease.

Answers	Total and %
Never	-
Rarely during the week	1 (0.57%)
Half the time during the week	5 (2.84%)
Occasionally during the week	12 (6.82%)
Often throughout the week	82 (46.59%)
Every day of the week	76 (43.18%)
Total	176 (100%)

Table 14. I have achieved useful things through my work.

Answers	Total and %
Never	0
Few times	6 (3.41%)
Almost always	112 (63.64%)
Always	58 (32.95%)
Total	176 (100%)

Table 15. Working with people is a source of satisfaction.

Answers	Total and %
Never	0
Rarely during the week	3 (1.7%)
Half the time during the week	17 (9.66%)
Occasionally during the week	18 (10.23%)
Often throughout the week	57 (32.38%)
Every day of the week	81 (46%)
Total	176 (100%)

Table 16. Working all day with people exhausts me.

Answers	Total and %
Never	23 (13.07%)
Rarely during the week	56 (31.82%)
Half the time during the week	20 (11.36%)
Occasionally during the week	28 (15.91%)
Often throughout the week	41 (23.29%)
Every day of the week	8 (4.54%)
Total	176 (100%)

6. Discussion of Results

From the interviews submitted to healthcare workers who work in contact with diabetic patients, we found that there was not a clear position on the presence of gender inequality in the work environment. Although some related aspects were particularly felt by the interviewees (for example, the majority of prestigious positions being held by men, or the disagreement with wage disparity). The data show that interviewees who perceived the presence of gender inequality in their company often felt fatigued by their work during the week and experienced anxiety and concern. In general, the state of anxiety and lack of motivation by some interviewees was attributed in part to the presence of gender inequality. However, the relationship with the patient seemed to be in most cases profitable, effective, and a source of satisfaction for most respondents. Healthcare workers were satisfied with working in contact with people and being part of their care path. The reasons why healthcare workers may experience situations of malaise in the workplace can be different (this includes gender inequality, personal hardships, the physical structures where they work, etc.). In the same way, the possible solutions and models through which organizations can promote all those factors that directly or indirectly affect the well-being and motivation of healthcare workers and can remove or decrease those negative effects are disparate. Promoting the well-being of healthcare workers in general, but especially for those working with chronic illnesses such as diabetes, improves the patient–healthcare worker relationship and allows healthcare workers to express their full potential by putting the patient at the center of care and allowing them to better cope with their illness.

7. Limits of Research and Future Studies

The phenomenon of gender inequality is very complex and occurs in different forms and nuances, depending upon the environment, people, and social context. The results presented relate to a small sample of respondents working in different geographical areas. Extending the survey to a larger number of respondents would allow for a more detailed and comprehensive analysis in order to study which variables might directly or indirectly affect the patient–healthcare worker relationship.

Author Contributions: Conceptualization, T.L.; methodology, T.L.; formal analysis, T.L.; investigation, T.L., S.C. and C.P.; data care, S.C.; preparation of the original draft, T.L., S.C. and C.P.; revision and modification, T.L., S.C. and C.P. All authors have read and agreed to the published version of the manuscript.

Funding: This research received no external funding.

Institutional Review Board Statement: Not applicable.

Informed Consent Statement: Not applicable.

Data Availability Statement: Not applicable.

Conflicts of Interest: The authors declare no conflict of interest.

References

1. Educazione Terapeutica Strutturata Nella Gestione Della Patologia Diabetica. Available online: https://www.siditalia.it/images/Documenti/Gised/49%20%20%20%20documento.pdf (accessed on 19 March 2022).
2. Renders, C.M.; Valk, G.D.; Griffin, S.J.; Wagner, E.H.; Eijk Van, J.T.; Assendelft, W.J. Interventions to Improve the Management of Diabetes in Primary Care, Outpatient, and Community Settings: A Systematic Review. *Diabetes Care* **2001**, *24*, 1821–1833. [CrossRef] [PubMed]
3. Skovlund, S.E.; Peyrot, M. The Diabetes Attitudes, Wishes, and Needs (DAWN) Program: A New Approach to Improving Outcomes of Diabetes Care. *Diabetes Spectr.* **2005**, *18*, 136–142. [CrossRef]
4. Morrison, F.; Shubina, M.; Goldberg, S.; Turchin, A. Performance of Primary Care Physicians and Other Providers on Key Process Measures in the Treatment of Diabetes. *Diabetes Care* **2012**, *36*, 1147–1152. [CrossRef] [PubMed]
5. WHO | World Health Organization. Available online: https://www.who.int/activities/value-gender-and-equity-in-the-global-health-workforce (accessed on 19 March 2022).
6. Gender Inequality | European Institute for Gender Equality. Available online: https://eige.europa.eu/thesaurus/terms/1182 (accessed on 19 March 2022).
7. Women in Global Health | Challenging Power and Privilege. Available online: https://www.womeningh.org/single-post/2019/11/06/whs-2019-gender-equality-within-the-global-health-workforce (accessed on 19 March 2022).
8. Global Gender Gap Report 2021 | World Economic Forum. Available online: https://www.weforum.org/reports/global-gender-gap-report-2021/ (accessed on 19 March 2022).
9. Tackling the Gender Pay Gap: Not without a Better Work-Life Balance | European Institute for Gender Equality. Available online: https://eige.europa.eu/publications/tackling-gender-pay-gap-not-without-better-work-life-balance (accessed on 19 March 2022).
10. Bottaro, C. Il ruolo dell'educatore professionale all'interno di un'equipe multidisciplinare nella presa in carico di pazienti affetti da diabete di diabete di tipo 2. *J. Health Care Educ. Pract.* **2020**, *10*, 79–80. [CrossRef]
11. Ciaccio, S.; Valentini, U. Il ruolo dell'educazione terapeutica nella cronicità. *MeDia* **2011**, *11*, 139–144.
12. Serrano-Gil, M.; Jacob, S. Engaging and empowering patients to manage their type 2 diabetes, Part I: A knowledge, attitudes, and practice gap? *Adv. Ther.* **2010**, *27*, 321–333. [CrossRef] [PubMed]
13. Agrusta, M.; By Berardino, P.; Gentile, L.; Visalli, N.; Bufacchi, T.; Gelfusa, F.; Pomilla, A.; Aglialoro, A.; Key, A.; Cipolloni, L.; et al. L'approccio 329 bio-psicosociale e la persona con diabete: Proposta di cartella educativa in diabetologia. *Il G. AMD* **2012**, *15*, 190–194.
14. Moretto, B. Educazione terapeutica del paziente tra competenze e contesti di cura: Riflessioni sul ruolo dell'educatore profes-331 sionale. *J. Health Care Educ. Pract.* **2019**, *1*, 1–15. [CrossRef]

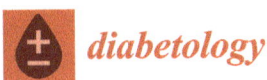

Article

Sex/Gender Psychological Differences in the Adult Diabetic Patient and How a Child's Response to Chronic Disease Varies with Age and Can Be Influenced by Technology

Maria Antonietta Taras [1],* and Alessandra Pellegrini [2],†

1. Diabetes and Metabolic Diseases Unit, 07026 Olbia, Italy
2. Freelance Psychologist and Psychotherapist, 90121 Palermo, Italy; alinacpellegrini@gmail.com
* Correspondence: anto.ta@inwind.it
† On behalf of the SIMDO working group of Psycology.

Citation: Taras, M.A.; Pellegrini, A. Sex/Gender Psychological Differences in the Adult Diabetic Patient and How a Child's Response to Chronic Disease Varies with Age and Can Be Influenced by Technology. *Diabetology* **2021**, *2*, 215–225. https://doi.org/10.3390/diabetology2040019

Academic Editor: Giancarlo Tonolo

Received: 2 September 2021
Accepted: 11 October 2021
Published: 1 November 2021

Publisher's Note: MDPI stays neutral with regard to jurisdictional claims in published maps and institutional affiliations.

Copyright: © 2021 by the authors. Licensee MDPI, Basel, Switzerland. This article is an open access article distributed under the terms and conditions of the Creative Commons Attribution (CC BY) license (https://creativecommons.org/licenses/by/4.0/).

Abstract: Chronic diseases have a negative impact on quality of life and perceived well-being. Depression tends to be more frequent in people with chronic diseases than the general population, and, for example, in diabetes, it has an incidence of two to three times higher and often remains under-diagnosed. The inability to control and predict the course of the disease exposes chronic patients to mood fluctuations which are often difficult to manage, also in virtue of the fact that in any chronic pathology a stabilization aimed at attenuating the symptoms or slowing the course is pursued, but it cannot tend to achieve complete healing. This fact of incurability for many subjects means the loss of control over their own body, in which the social and family role is also perceived as compromised and the experienced distress can result in the appearance of underlying disorders, both psychological or psychiatric. In this area, there is currently a great deal of focus on sex/gender differences. The aim of this article is to highlight these differences with regard to the emotional aspects that most affect the management of diabetic pathology. In this paper, we will underline a particularly underestimated eating disorder: diabulimia, then that the perception of itself is not only related to the sex assigned at birth, but also to the gender that is acquired during life, and we will also analyze the three phases related to the acquisition of gender identity during the evolutionary period. Finally, we will talk about the use of technology in diabetic patients (insulin pumps, continuous glucose monitoring variably integrated into each other) that might generate a series of psychological–behavioral reactions related to the integration between technology and body image and the experience of social acceptance of the individual, particularly in the evolution age.

Keywords: anxiety; depression; diabulimia; developmental age

The Emotional Aspects Affecting Diabetes in Adult (M.A. Taras)

1. Introduction

Diabetes mellitus and cardiovascular diseases act like two sides of the same coin: diabetes is considered as an equivalent of ischemic cardiovascular disease while patients with ischemic cardiovascular disease often have diabetes or pre-diabetes. The two major forms of diabetes are type 1 insulin-dependent diabetes (T1DM) and type 2 non-insulin-dependent diabetes (T2DM). Although we are interested in diabetes, the premises are in common with other chronic diseases. All chronic diseases have a negative impact on the quality of life and perceived well-being, the uncertain and unpredictable development of the disease exposes from the outset to a higher incidence of anxiety and mood disorders such as depression, which tends to be more frequent in these subjects than in the general population [1]. In diabetes, depression has an incidence two to three times higher and very often remains under-diagnosed [2]. There is evidence that the prevalence of depression is moderately increased in prediabetic patients and in undiagnosed diabetic patients, and markedly increased in the previously diagnosed diabetic patients compared to normal glucose metabolism individuals [2]. On the other hand, depression may increase the risk of developing type 2 diabetes by 60% [3,4]. It seems that there is a bidirectional association between diabetes and depression, a complex relationship that might share biological mechanisms, whose understanding could provide better treatment and improve the outcomes for these pathologies. In diabetic patients, depression remains under-diagnosed and an important aspect for the diabetic specialist would be the awareness of this quite common co-morbidity. Risk factors such as negative body image, perceived poor state of well-being, difficulty in daily management towards dietary and pharmacological therapy significantly alters the quality of life and when coping skills are lacking distress will results, creating a suffering experience that can generate depressive symptoms and/or in a real depression. These factors show differences in sex/gender and a different impact in the different stages of life. Women are surely more affected than men: in adolescence eating disorders and in adulthood the worst perception of quality of life are among the factors most heartfelt. A multidisciplinary approach of the diabetic patient would help to improve the outcomes of both diseases, decreasing the number of DALYs (disability-adjusted life years) and even mortality.

The inability to control and predict the course and outcomes of chronic disease exposes patients to mood fluctuations which are often difficult to manage in which the periods of relative well-being allow a greater adaptive response. On the contrary, during the exacerbation of symptoms, the quality of life is affected, leading to developing emotional symptoms fed by a course that cannot tend to complete healing but only stabilize the symptoms or eventually slow them down. This for many patients means the loss of control over their own body, to which an experience of frustration is added where their social and family role is perceived as a compromise because family members are heavily involved in the management of the disease. This would increase the sense of impotence that, in many patients, could cause a psychological maladaptive response with activation of defense mechanisms where the disease is scotomized, resulting in poor compliance or even turning into subthreshold psychological disorders, or even psychiatric. Emotional vulnerability shows gender peculiarities and more attention is paid now to these differences than in the past. There is general agreement that women suffer from depression two to three times more than men.

2. Sex/Gender Definition

Regarding sex and gender, we must do a clarification: gender is a social construct operating at all ages from the fetus in intrauterine ambient to the elderly, that generally transforms a female into a woman and a male into a man, giving the different roles, relationships and the different access to education and occupation attributed to women and men, irrespective of their genetic make-up at the chromosomal level, whereas sex is the biological/hormonal aspect of male and female derived by the presence of chromosomes XX or XY, since the two concepts are jointed and difficult to dissect we will use the term sex/gender from now on as previously suggested by others [5]. The mechanisms underlying the development of certain diseases in women are studied today more than in the past because for long-time women were "de facto" excluded from clinical trials due to the need to use sometimes complex birth control systems in order to avoid pregnancies with new drugs.

3. Sex/Gender Differences in Diabetes

Regarding sex/gender clinical differences in diabetes and even in the prediabetic state, nowadays there is several pieces of evidence, although a lot is still controversial either in the response to drugs and in the pathophysiological evolution and chronic complications of the disease. For more details that elude the purpose of this work, we refer to some fairly recent reviews on the subject [5–7].

Despite the delay, now we have data showing different gender behaviors that affect different management, in which metabolic control and age also significantly influence the psychosocial response to the disease [8,9]. These differences have also emerged in communication exchanges, thanks to which behaviors and emotions are expressed. There are different sex/gender inclinations in which women tend to manifest their emotions more openly, have strong relational dispositions and show a greater empathic capacity. Despite their multitasking abilities, they show a greater vulnerability to the emotional sphere, and, compared to men, women more easily require help, which may justify the increased prevalence of disorders. In diabetes, it can be observed that despite sudden glycemic changes that affect both sexes, significantly complicating compliance to drug and life behavior indications, the social role played by women (family duties, work) probably leads to neglect of the disease that then becomes an individual responsibility with the emotions tending to be more negative, despite greater efforts in the management and a better knowledge of pathology, resulting in a life of less social support, while in men the management of diabetes takes place more in the family context. In real life, a Korean study explored the relationship between T2DM and employment status, suggesting a greater negative influence of T2DM in women than in men [10]. The role played by the emotional aspects has been well studied, but it is still a topic of debate. There is no agreement between clinicians whether anxiety and mood disorders in diabetes precede diabetes or are the consequence of it. A positive attitude and acceptance towards the pathology lead to greater perceived well-being and this reverberates positively in the management of diabetes. In fact, the close connection between the endocrine and limbic systems causes some emotional states, including anxiety, which promotes the release of adrenaline and cortisol that hinder the action of insulin and consequently cause hyperglycemia. Psychiatric disorders and diabetes also share a bidirectional association, influencing each other in several ways; compared to control groups, diabetic patients have a worse quality of life, depressive disorders and anxiety disorders [11] and have a double chance of incurring a depressive episode compared to non-diabetic subjects [12,13]. Therefore, having diabetes and being a woman can significantly increase the risk of having a major depressive disorder [14]. People with diabetes of both sexes are also more likely to suffer from anxiety disorders than non-diabetic people [15]. A Canadian study examined the association between anxiety symptoms and physical inactivity in T2DM diabetic patients aged 40 to 75 years (over a follow up of ten years). It was found that the symptoms of anxiety are significant clinical comorbidities and men, in this case, may represent a particularly vulnerable subgroup [16]. Compared to the quality of life, in a study on a random cohort of T1DM adult diabetics, adult women with long-standing T1DM showed the lower quality of life, probably related to higher frequency and severity of psychopathological syndromes [17]. Additionally, the age of onset seems to show differences, since T1DM women with childhood-onset have greater distress in general [18].

4. Eating Disorders

The vulnerability of diabetic patients to different psychological conditions does not allow them to reach adequate levels of compliance and, among these, eating disorders (ED) have also taken on particular importance, precisely because of the consequences in the management of the disease. The real extent of the association between diabetes and ED is still under-estimated and shows peculiarities with anorexia nervosa, bulimia, and uncontrolled ED. The literature reports that the diagnosis of diabetes can lead to the development of ED in T1DM diabetics while in T2DM it seems to be already antecedent to the diagnosis [19], compared to the general population, ED appears to be more frequent in type 1 diabetics. Regarding anorexia nervosa, there are no significant differences in the prevalence in people with T1DM compared to controls whereas in women, a higher prevalence of bulimia is present [20]. A systematic review carried out on electronic databases and meta-analysis found a higher prevalence of alterations in food behavior in adolescents with T1DM diabetes (39.3%) compared to controls (32.5%) and this was associated with lower blood sugar control [21]. A multicenter study on the comorbidities between T1DM and T2DM and ED showed no differences in ED prevalence rates in both types of diabetes with different features of ED distribution, bulimia being more prevalent in T1DM, while binge eating in T2DM. The results show that neither ED nor omission of insulin therapy is necessarily associated with poor blood sugar control [22]. Our interest in ED is mainly in relation to a particular form of dietary behavior: diabulimia, the term of which comes from the words diabetes and bulimia, consisting in the arbitrary reduction or omission of insulin, the result of which is an abrupt rise in blood sugar, in which there is a massive loss of glucose with urine (glycosuria) with calorie loss which also results in rapid weight loss exposing to the risk of ketoacidosis [23]. It was identified by a group of British physicians in around 2009 who observed that a number of T1DM diabetic patients, predominantly female, did not properly handle the prescribed insulin doses: this can be defined as a subtype of ED [24]. There is no consistent explanation for the origin of the disturbance. As for ED in the general population, this type of disorder shows sex/gender differences: it is more frequent in the female sex and increases with age, with a prevalence that can reach up to 40% of young adults with T1DM [25]. The chronic nature of the disease has additional risk factors that would favor its development, such as poor self-image, the constant attention to diet and the action of insulin on weight gain, factors that contribute synergistically and condition the course leading to extreme choices such as precisely reducing or omitting insulin to achieve the ideal weight [26]. In one study, the intentional omission affected about 31% of women of all ages but only 8,8% reported frequent omissions [27].

An unexplained metabolic imbalance can be considered as a wake-up call to which clinicians should pay more attention as the phenomenon is growing. This disease in diabetes is still very undervalued, partly because the tests available for the diagnosis of the disorder do not take into account that in diabetes, the diet has a fundamental role and excessive attention to the same may be the cause of the exacerbation of the disorder. In addition, in the Diabetes Units often there are no specific professional skills, such as psychologists, that through the use of clinical tests and interviews can bring to light this type of problem, that if not properly investigated could run into false diagnosis. In a study aimed at investigating whether in women with T1DM insulin restriction led to an increase in morbidity and mortality, compared to other psychological distress, in an 11-year follow-up study in 234 women with T1DM, authors found that deceased women reported more significant ED symptoms ($p < 0.05$) and a more frequent insulin restriction ($p < 0.05$) at baseline as compared to survived women [28]. In this regard, we recently conducted a survey in our Diabetic Unit, aimed at assessing the presence of generic disorders of dietary behavior in a diabetic population in intensive insulin treatment consisting of T1DM and T2DM with at least four insulin injections a day, divided by gender and age. We administered the DEPS-R questionnaire anonymously [29] in two ways: in-person while waiting for the visit in the clinic and online via a spreadsheet that can be filled in on the website "www.janasdia.com" accessed on 10 October 2020. The analysis of the data shows no differences between the two routes of administration of the questionnaire and therefore the results were analyzed in their entirety: n = 410 diabetic patients in intensive insulin therapy with four injections/day (Table 1: T1DM = 314; T2DM = 96). The DEPS-R questionnaire is considered positive when the total score is equal to/more than 22. The score is obtained from the sum of the answers, where never = 0 while always = 5. In addition to considering the test in its completeness, were also analyzed the answers to some questions particularly addressed the failure to administer insulin voluntarily, namely questions number 4, 9, 11, 13 and 16. The female sex showed a significant prevalence on the male sex ($p = 0.049$) in the overall sample in reaching the positive quorum of 22, this trend was maintained after dividing the subjects in T1DM and T2DM. The positive T2DM subjects did not differ in age and duration of diabetes compared to the negative ones, while in positive T1DM male subjects had a significant ($p = 0.018$) age difference, belonging on average to the most advanced age groups (over 40 years). In addition, by analyzing the scores of the answers to the questions in their entirety, the female sex confirmed both in

T1DM and in T2DM, a score in its entirety significantly higher, which remained positive in T1DM (0.0447) and T2DM (0.049), see Table 1. By analyzing the scores for the most significant questions related to diabulimia, the female sex presented a score significantly higher than the male ($p = 0.0172$) in T2DM for question 9 "I try to keep my blood sugar high so that I will lose weight" and for question 11 "I feel fat when I take all of my insulin" in T1DM 1 ($p = 0.0004$), while no significant differences were evident for the other applications. Regarding the more specific question 8, "I make myself vomiting" a total of 17 people with no sex differences responded positively, but with a higher prevalence in T1DM (T1DM: F = 5, M = 8; T2DM: F = 2, M = 2). Our research confirms that there are eating disorders below the threshold in a not negligible prevalence in diabetic patients without large differences between type 1 and 2, but with clear sex/gender differences.

Table 1. Results DPRS-R test in T1DM and T2DM divided for sex.

	Diabetes			
	T1DM		T2DM	
	M	F	M	F
N = 410	133	181	44	52
Age (years) Mean ± SD	28 ± 6 *	27 ± 7 *	58 ± 9	62 ± 10
DPRS-R SCORE ≥ 22, n (%)	8 (6%)	20 (11%)	9 (21%)	19 (36%)
p	$p = 0.0447$		$p = 0.049$	

Data in Table 1 represent the four groups studied: male and female T1DM and male and female T2DM: numbers in each group, as well as mean age± SD of the different groups and the number (%) of positive answers to DPRS-R test with statistical significance, is also given. To determine if the means of the sets of data regarding age were significantly different from each other we used the independent (unpaired) samples t-test, while Pearson Chi-squared test were used to test differences in % positive answers to DPRS-R score. T1DM = type 1 insulin-dependent diabetes, T2DM = type 2 insulin-independent, but insulin-treated patients, M = male, F = female, n = number. * $p < 0.01$ T1DM vs. T2DM, male vs. female within each group were not significantly different for age. Pearson Chi-square revealed significant differences between males and females within each group of diabetic patients, without differences between the two different kinds of diabetes.

5. Patient and Care Provider Dyads

Last but not least important we must remember that compliance to drug treatment and lifestyle changes implies of course patient and care provider collaboration, thus emphasizing the role of patient and care provider dyads. Nevertheless, guidelines do not deeply consider the sex/gender of care providers, forgetting that he/she is a person, and every individual is sexed and gendered. However, the importance of care provider sex/gender is emerging and its influence on health quality has been known for a long time [30,31]. During communication training, these differences should be taken into account, especially to strengthen male communication skills and improve their attitudes [32], since it appears evident that physician gender influences quality of care in patients with type 2 diabetes, with female physicians providing overall better quality of care, especially in prognostic important risk factors management [33]. It was suggested that the influence of sex/gender on adherence appears particularly important, thus programs aimed to address men- and women-specific needs are recommended to increase adherence in both sexes, paying attention also to caregiver–patient dyads [34].

6. Conclusions First Part

In this first part, we mainly analyzed the psychological aspects related to the differences in sex/gender in diabetes in adulthood. Particular attention was given to eating disorders that are present as a subsoil condition in diabetic disease with a prevalence not suspected in the past. These disorders may be pre-existing to diabetic disease or they might be the consequence of a number of restrictions mainly food, imposed by the diabetic disease.

Now we will analyze the paths that can lead to the definition of gender during the various stages of growth, an important chapter to better define the mechanisms in adulthood. A chapter will also address the possible psychological impact that technologies may have in the development of gender differences inherent in the acceptance of the diabetic disease.

7. The Acquisition of Itself during Evolution (A. Pellegrini)

The Three Phases Relating to the Acquisition of Gender Identity during Childhood

As already pointed out, the term gender expresses the social meaning assumed by sexual differences, it represents the constellation of elements and behaviors associated with males and females and therefore expected from them within the community. Gender identity is the result of a process of identity construction that begins in early childhood and continues throughout life, assuming stability only in the post-adolescent era. Speaking of gender identity means referring to the perception that the subject has of himself and it is not comparable to the mere sex of belonging assigned at birth [35]. During childhood, three phases, relating to the acquisition of gender identity, can be identified [36,37]:

- **Gender membership:** Children from the age of two are able to discriminate whether they are male or female.
- **Gender stability:** Children from 4 years of age realize that the sex of a person remains unchanged for life.
- **Gender perseverance:** children aged 6/7 years recognize their gender identity even if not matched with their physical appearance.

Several studies highlight the importance of the quality of the child's first emotional relationships while taking into high consideration the multifactorial aspects that affect the development of the self and gender identity [37,38]. A child's response to chronic disease varies with age. As early as 1930 Anna Freud [39] had highlighted how physical illness could have consequences on the psychological development of the child, especially if it lasted a long time. Hospitalization and prolonged care could interrupt or interfere in the very delicate evolutionary process of the child with different consequences related to the age of onset of the disease, its severity, its duration. In this regard, in fact, it is important to recognize and understand the reciprocal effects between chronic disease and the process of maturation. Given the fact that any chronic disease can interfere, in a transitory or permanent way, with the physiological processes of maturation and development, in the same manner, the opposite can happen, that is physiological transformations, and consequently, psychosocial adaptations can have a positive or negative influence on the natural history of a disease. In a study conducted in a Pediatric Diabetes Center in southern Italy, the psychological problems and self-perception of a sample of 81 children with Type 1 Diabetes Mellitus (T1DM) were assessed. A graphic test was used, the drawing of the human figure according to the "Draw a Person procedure: Screening Procedure for Emotional Disturbances". It was found that children with diabetes drew the smallest human figures, highlighting aspects of the body image different from those of the healthy control group. However, no gender differences emerged. The results support the need to monitor the characteristics of the perception of body image in children with T1DM during their development course, in order to prevent the onset of psychological discomfort.

On the other hand, health facilities today appear and tend to be more organized and responsive to the needs of patients in developmental age with chronic diseases. The management of the chronic disease requires special skills on the part of the doctor who takes care of young patients, the latter should possess, in addition to the specific skills of the actual pathology, knowledge of the psychological and social aspects of the subject and his family. This cognitive need is maintained when the patient is an adolescent. During this phase of growth, the question of identity assumes a central value, being the phase of the redefinition of the self and self-image. The non-negligible role of the body, which is central in the psychic development of the individual, in this period, assumes a greater resonance, in a rapid and sudden way the body is transformed, taking on strange, disharmonious appearances that procure new and disturbing sensations in a mind that is in part anchored to infantile functioning. These transformations set up a real emotional storm which the subject must come face to face with and have to integrate into his own psyche. The adolescent experience goes through moments of uncertainty, sadness, fear and this condition can determine the appearance of negative feelings towards oneself and towards one's perception as being responsible for having generated a non-perfect body. Dissatisfaction can evolve in forms of discomfort: self-injurious behaviors and acting out, drastic diets, depression, isolation and so on. This delicate phase can become even more so when you have a chronic disease. The disease affects the body and is a source of physical and mental suffering. It generates experiences and defensive mechanisms, and in some cases, it becomes a constant in everyday life, causing changes in daily habits. The condition of T1DM significantly affects and influences the life habits of the subject and, therefore, everyone, but in particular, the adolescent may show a certain difficulty in emotional adaptation to the disease, reacting in some ways: anger, denial of the disease, sense of injustice, amplification of the negative aspects of the disease, identification with one's own disease, an association of diabetes with all difficult complex and negative experiences, feeling of diversity.

The optimal control of diabetes at this stage of development represents a "problem" for the adolescent himself, for his family and for the diabetes team taking care of him. Gender differences can influence the doctor–patient relationship in the treatment path. It is therefore necessary that the specialist doctor, in addition to being competent in his discipline, knows the bases of the emotional-affective-relational development of the individual so that he can understand the resonances in the therapeutic path. The scientific literature shows that male adolescents are more prone to agitation and impulsiveness than females who show greater criticality in the emotional dimension and body perception. The diabetic adolescent can experience strong emotions as a function of the dilemma experienced within himself, generated by the solicitations coming from the peer group, that sometimes push in the opposite direction to the choices that in reality, he should make as more appropriate for his health. In the diabetic adolescent, this conflict and the natural defiant behavior, expression of the desire for perception and identification of the limit, could have a negative impact on the correct execution of insulin therapy, for example being the cause of delay or non-intake of the same. In girls, on the other hand, the obligatory attention to nutrition could stimulate or amplify issues related to physical appearance and weight control, the effects of which could negatively reflect on the remodeling of insulin therapy or could create the basis for the development of an eating disorder. Sometimes there is a delay in the age of menarche in girls, especially if the onset of diabetes occurred in the first puberty, this could have psychological effects and consequences. At the conclusion of a study [40], whose goal was to investigate age at menarche in young women withT1DM and examine the effect of diabetes management (HbA1c level, number of blood glucose checks, insulin therapy intensity, and insulin dose) on age at menarche, in those diagnosed before menarche (about 300 very young T1DM girls) it emerged that the mean age at menarche is greater than the mean age of the non-diabetic, although the distance in time is reduced as better glycemic control is achieved. Ages at menarche and diagnosis were not associated. For those diagnosed before menarche, age at menarche was delayed 1.3 months with each 1% increase in mean total HbA1c level in the 3 years before menarche.

8. Gender Dysphoria

Another important issue in adolescence is gender dysphoria (suffering that results from the inconsistency between gender and gender identity). Adolescents with gender dysphoria are described as the most psychologically and socially vulnerable population. It is a condition that is associated with profound psychological suffering and the associated psychopathologies seem to have their onset or strengthen at the same time as pubertal development since at this moment there is a confrontation with a body that changes in an unwanted direction. In a very recent publication [41] the authors studied the prevalence of gender dysphoria (GD) in youth given the fact that environmental triggers, such as psychological minority stress experienced by youth with GD, may influence the management of T1DM (10 to 21 years) with important clinical implications. The objective of this study was to determine the prevalence of concurrent diagnosis of T1DM and GD in adolescents evaluated at a university-based children's hospital. Data were collected for 749,284 individual patients during the review period (ten years follow-up). There were 2017 patients diagnosed with T1DM for a prevalence rate of 2.69 per 1000 and 315 patients diagnosed with GD for a prevalence rate of 0.42 per 1000. Concurrent diagnosis of both T1DM and GD was found in eight patients. The prevalence rate for T1DM in the non-GD population is 2.68 (95% CI 2.57–2.80) per 1000 vs. 24.77 (95% CI: 12.60–48.10) per 1000 in the GD population ($p < 0.0001$). The prevalence of T1DM in the population of adolescents diagnosed with GD is 9.4-fold higher (95% CI: 4.7–19.1, $p < 0.0001$) than the prevalence rate of T1DM alone in the overall adolescent patient group. Glycemic control initially improved after the first GD clinic visit over a mean interval of 5 months but was not sustained. There was no improvement in HbA1c in those that initiated puberty blocker therapy and gender-affirming hormone therapy. Stress reduction due to initiation of gender-affirming hormone therapy could lead to short-term improvement in diabetes control in adolescents with T1DM and GD. Glycemic control in T1DM often worsens during adolescence due to puberty-related insulin resistance and treatment adherence in T1DM often declines during adolescence (decrease in parental oversight and an increase in the prevalence of psychiatric comorbidities). For those adolescents with T1DM and GD who have established a trusting relationship with their diabetes team it could be more comfortable discussing gender identity and may be more likely to seek medical care related to gender identity. Lack of such a relationship with health care providers can impede or delay the diagnosis of GD. In a study [42] conducted at Oslo University Hospital in Norway, on a sample of 105 adolescents with T1DM, (12–20 years) of which 44 males and 61 females, 65.3% were insulin pump users and 33.7% on multiple daily insulin injections therapy. Among this population, significant gender differences were observed in disease perception, insulin concern, and social and family coping strategies. The results of the study showed that females had significantly higher negative perceptions of their T1DM than males on all of the Brief Illness Perception Questionnaire (BIPQ) items ($p < 0.05$). Females instead scored significantly higher than males on insulin concern ($p < 0.001$), indicating more negative perceptions/more concerns about insulin. Males and females did not significantly differ in their perceptions of insulin necessity. There were no statistically significant differences in insulin beliefs between patients treated with insulin pumps versus the pen. Patients using an insulin pen had however significantly more negative views on treatment control than patients using pumps, respectively ($p < 0.05$). With regard to the subscales, females scored significantly higher on being social and solving family problems (both p's < 0.01), indicating more positive coping among females than males for these subscales. There were no statistically significant differences in coping strategies between patients treated with insulin pumps versus a pen. In conclusion, the study highlights how the management of psychological aspects can be a clinically important supplement to the treatment of T1DM and that a tailored therapeutic approach for males and females can be justified.

9. Psychological Aspect of Technology in Diabetic Patients

Regarding the possible influence of technology in diabetes, we must consider that the use of the insulin pump and/or sensor for continuous glucose monitoring could generate a series of psychological-behavioral reactions related to the integration between it and the body image and the experience of social acceptance of the individual. The impact that the insulin pump has on body image is also affected by gender differences [43]:

- Adolescent females express this impact more and express their concern regarding the integration of a mechanical device into their own body; their uncertainties are

expressed in terms of perception of the insulin pump as an external or internal presence in one's body.
- Adolescents males have less concern and less hesitation with respect to social approval in relation to the use of the insulin pump.

Age, male gender, and social deprivation are still associated with a lower rate of insulin pump therapy initiation at least in adults with T1DM and it is well established that an improved clinical outcome is associated with the early initiation of insulin pump therapy in children with type 1 diabetes [44]. The psychological aspect of sex/gender difference must be taken into account in order to optimize pump therapy and the other technological devices such as continuous glucose monitoring in these patients. Since the impact that "technology" has on body image is affected by gender differences, the management of psychological aspects is a clinically important supplement to a tailored therapeutic approach for males and females.

In light of the foregoing, the help and support provided to adolescents in this phase of development and criticality can lead to a positive effect and the success of the treatment process. At the same time, they influence the process of raising awareness of the state of health. The relationship is an integral part of the treatment process and, above all, in the case of chronic illness, it is much more of a powerful tool that facilitates the involvement of the adolescent facilitating and strengthening the latter's ability to draw on inner resources to be able to creatively coexist with his pathology. In the relationship of care and help, one must know how to accept, listen and put the other at ease, managing to keep the right distance and, at the same time, showing empathy. It is necessary to assist and accompany the adolescent in this phase of transition, to recognize and pay attention to his symptoms as alarm bells and to help him towards empowerment.

10. Key Messages (M.A.Taras)

At the end of this manuscript we can say that the psychological aspects of chronic diseases, such as diabetes, play an important role in the evolution of the disease and its management, ultimately with repercussions on compliance to drug and lifestyle modifications. These aspects, which vary according to sex/gender and age, as well as the context in which the patient lives, require psychologists trained in chronic diseases who should be part of the diabetologist team.

Author Contributions: Conceptualization, M.A.T. and A.P.; methodology, M.A.T. and A.P.; resources, M.A.T. and A.P.; writing—original draft preparation, M.A.T. and A.P.; writing—review and editing, M.A.T. and A.P. M.A.T. and A.P. contributed equally to the paper been in charge of respective chapters as indicated by the names. All authors have read and agreed to the published version of the manuscript.

Funding: This research received no external funding.

Institutional Review Board Statement: Not applicable.

Informed Consent Statement: Not applicable.

Data Availability Statement: Not applicable.

Acknowledgments: We want to thank all the patients who voluntarily responded to the DEPS-R questionnaire.

Conflicts of Interest: The authors declare no conflict of interest in this paper.

References

1. Evans, D.L.; Charney, D.S. Mood Disorders and medical illness: A major public health problem. *Biol. Psychiatry* **2003**, *54*, 177–180. [CrossRef]
2. Bădescu, S.V.; Tătaru, C.; Kobylinska, L.; Georgescu, E.L.; Zahiu, D.M.; Zăgrean, A.M.; Zăgrean, L. The association between Diabetes mellitus and Depression. *J. Med. Life* **2016**, *9*, 120–126.
3. Mezuk, B.; Eaton, W.W.; Albrecht, S.; Golden, S.H. Depression and type 2 diabetes over the lifespan: A meta-analysis. *Diabetes Care* **2008**, *31*, 2383–2390. [CrossRef] [PubMed]

4. Rubin, R.R.; Ma, Y.; Marrero, D.G.; Peyrot, M.; Barrett-Connor, E.L.; Kahn, S.E.; Haffner, S.M.; Price, D.W.; Knowler, W.C. Elevated depression symptoms, antidepressant medicine use, and risk of developing diabetes during the diabetes prevention program. *Diabetes Care* **2008**, *31*, 420–426. [CrossRef]
5. Franconi, F.; Campesi, I.; Occhioni, S.; Tonolo, G. Sex-gender differences in diabetes vascular complications and treatment. *Endocr. Metab. Immune Disord. Drug Targets* **2012**, *12*, 179–196. [CrossRef]
6. Seghieri, G.; Policardo, L.; Anichini, R.; Franconi, F.; Campesi, I.; Cherchi, S.; Tonolo, G. The Effect of Sex and Gender on Diabetic Complications. *Curr. Diabetes Rev.* **2017**, *13*, 148–160. [CrossRef] [PubMed]
7. Campesi, I.; Occhioni, S.; Tonolo, G.; Cherchi, S.; Basili, S.; Carru, C.; Zinellu, A.; Franconi, F. Ageing/Menopausal status in healthy women and aging healthy men differently affect cardiometabolic parameters. *Int. J. Med. Sci.* **2016**, *13*, 124–132. [CrossRef]
8. Siddiqui, M.A.; Khan, M.F.; Carline, T.E. Gender Differences in Living with Diabetes Mellitus. *Mat. Soc. Med.* **2013**, *25*, 140–142. [CrossRef]
9. Kim, J.H.; Lee, W.Y.; Lee, S.S.; Kim, Y.T.; Hong, Y.P. Gender Differences in the Relationship between Type 2 Diabetes Mellitus and Employment: Evidence from the Korea Health Panel Study. *Int. J. Environ. Ris. Public Health* **2020**, *17*, 7040. [CrossRef]
10. Balhara, Y.P. Diabetes and psychiatric disorders. *Indian J Endocrinol. Metab.* **2011**, *15*, 274–283. [CrossRef]
11. Lustman, P.J.; Penckofer, S.M.; Clouse, R.E. Recent advances in understanding depression in adults with diabetes. *Curr. Psychiatry Per.* **2008**, *10*, 495–502. [CrossRef] [PubMed]
12. Eaton, W.W. Epidemiologic evidence on the comorbidity of depression and diabetes. *J. Psychosom. Res.* **2002**, *53*, 903–906. [CrossRef]
13. Anderson, R.J.; Freedland, K.E.; Clouse, R.E.; Lustman, P.J. The prevalence of comorbid depression in adults with diabetes: A meta-analysis. *Diabetes Care* **2001**, *24*, 1069–1078. [CrossRef]
14. Deischinger, C.; Dervic, E.; Leutner, M.; Kosi-Trebotic, L.; Klimek, P.; Kautzky, A.; Kautzky-Willer, A. Diabetes mellitus is associated with a higher risk for major depressive disorder in women than in men. *BMJ Open Diabetes Res. Care* **2020**, *8*, e001430. [CrossRef] [PubMed]
15. Vaghela, K.J. Anxiety among Diabetic and non Diabetic Male & Female. *Int. J. Indian Psychol.* **2016**, *3*, 76.
16. Lipscombe, C.; Smith, K.J.; Gariépy, G.; Schmitz, N. Gender differences in the relationship between anxiety symptoms and physical inactivity in a community-based sample of adults with type 2 diabetes. *Can. J. Diabetes* **2014**, *38*, 444–451. [CrossRef]
17. Castellano-Guerrero, A.M.; Guerrero, R.; Ruiz-Aranda, D.; Perea, S.; Pumar, A.; Relimpio, F.; Mangas, M.A.; Losada, F.; Martínez-Brocca, M.A. Gender differences in quality of life in adults with long-standing type 1 diabetes mellitus. *Diabetol. Metab. Syndr.* **2020**, *12*, 64. [CrossRef]
18. Lašaitė, L.; Ostrauskas, R.; Žalinkevičius, R.; Jurgevičienė, N.; Radzevičienė, L. Diabetes distress in adult type 1 diabetes mellitus men and women with disease onset in childhood and in adulthood. *J. Diabetes Complicat.* **2016**, *30*, 133–137. [CrossRef] [PubMed]
19. Gagnon, C.; Aimé, A.; Bélanger, C. Predictors of Comorbid Eating Disorders and Diabetes in People with Type 1 and Type 2 Diabetes. *Can. J. Diabetes* **2017**, *41*, 52–57. [CrossRef]
20. Mannucci, E.; Rotella, F.; Ricca, V.; Moretti, S.; Placidi, G.F.; Rotella, C.M. Eating disorders in patients with type 1 diabetes: A meta-analysis. *J. Endocrinol. Investig.* **2005**, *28*, 417–419. [CrossRef]
21. Young, V.; Eiser, C.; Johnson, B.; Brierley, S.; Epton, T.; Elliott, J.; Heller, S. Eating problems in adolescents with Type1 diabetes: A systematic review with meta-analysis. *Diabet. Med. A J. Br. Diabet. Assoc.* **2013**, *30*, 189–198. [CrossRef] [PubMed]
22. Herpertz, S.; Albus, C.; Wagener, R.; Kocnar, M.; Wagner, R.; Henning, A.; Migliore, F.; Foerster, H.; Schulze, S.B.; Thomas, W.; et al. Comorbidity of diabetes and eating disorders. Does diabetes control reflect disturbed eating behavior? *Diabetes Care* **1998**, *21*, 1110–1116. [CrossRef] [PubMed]
23. Tonolo, G.; Taras, M.A. Sex-Gender Difference in Diabetes: A Physiological and Psychological Point of View. *Women Health Complicat.* **2021**, *1*, 1–6.
24. Diabulimia. Available online: https://it.wikipedia.org/wiki/Diabulimia (accessed on 16 June 2021).
25. Pinhas-Hamiel, O.; Hamiel, U.; Levy-Shraga, Y. Eating disorders in adolescents with type 1 diabetes: Challenges in diagnosis and treatment. *World J. Diabetes* **2015**, *6*, 517–526. [CrossRef]
26. Baginsky, P. A patient's perspective A Battle to Overcome "Diabulimia" Commentary. *Am. Fam. Physician* **2009**, *79*, 263–268.
27. Polonsky, W.H.; Anderson, B.J.; Lohrer, P.A.; Aponte, J.E.; Jacobson, A.M.; Cole, C.F. Insulin omission in women with IDDMI. *Diabetes Care* **1994**, *17*, 1178–1185. [CrossRef] [PubMed]
28. Goebel-Fabbri, A.E.; Fikkan, J.; Franko, D.L.; Pearson, K.; Anderson, B.J.; Weinger, K. Insulin restriction and associated morbidity and mortality in women with type 1 diabetes. *Diabetes Care* **2008**, *31*, 415–419. [CrossRef]
29. Markowitz, J.T.; Butler, D.A.; Volkening, L.K.; Antsdei, J.E.; Anderson, B.J.; Laffei, L.M.B. Brief screening tool for disordered eating in diabetes. *Diabetes Care* **2010**, *33*, 495–500. [CrossRef] [PubMed]
30. Domenighetti, G.; Luraschi, P.; Marazzi, A. Hysterectomy and sex of the gynecologist. *NEJM* **1985**, *313*, 148–153.
31. Lurie, N.; Slater, J.; McGovern, P.; Ekstrum, J.; Quam, L.; Margolis, K. Preventive Care for women: Does the sex of the physician matter? *NEJM* **1993**, *329*, 478–482. [CrossRef]
32. Seitz, T.; Billeth, S.; Pastner, B.; Preusche, I.; Seidman, C. Significance of gender in the attitude towards doctor-patient communication in medical students and physicians. *Wien. Klin. Wochenschr.* **2016**, *128*, 663–668.

33. Berthold, H.K.; Gouni-Berthold, I.; Bestehorn, K.P.; Böhm, M.; Krone, W. Physician gender is associated with the quality of type 2 diabetes care. *J. Intern. Med.* **2008**, *264*, 340–350. [CrossRef] [PubMed]
34. Franconi, F.; Campesi, I. Sex and gender influences on pharmacological esponse: An overview. *Expert Rev. Clin. Pharmacol.* **2014**, 1–17.
35. Kjellberg, G. Acquiring a sexual identity. *Rev. Med. Suisse* **2013**, *9*, 606–609. [PubMed]
36. Meyer, J.K. The theory of gender identity disorders. *J. Am. Psychoanal. Assoc.* **1982**, *30*, 381–418. [CrossRef]
37. Malik, F.; Marwaha, R. Developmental Stages of Social Emotional Development. In *Children*; StatPearls Publishing: Treasure Island, FL, USA, 2021.
38. Hornor, G. Attachment Disorders. *J. Pediatr. Health Care* **2019**, *33*, 612–622. [CrossRef] [PubMed]
39. Freud, A. *Normality and Pathology in Childhood: Assessments of Development*; Routledge: London, UK, 1965.
40. Danielson, K.; Palta, M.; Allen, C.; D'Alessio, D.J. The Association of Increased Total Glycosylated Hemoglobin Levels with Delayed Age at Menarche in Young Women with T1DM. *J. Clin. Endocrinol. Metab.* **2005**, *90*, 6466–6471. [CrossRef]
41. Logel, S.N.; Bekx, M.T.; Rehm, J.L. Potential association between T1DMmellitus and gender dysphoria. *Pediatric Diabetes* **2020**, *21*, 266–270. [CrossRef]
42. Wisting, L.; Bang, L.; Skrivarhaug, T.; Dahl-Jørgensen, K.; Rø, Ø. Psychological barriers to optimal insulin therapy: More concerns in adolescent females than males. *BMJ Open Diabetes Res. Care.* **2016**, *4*, e000203. [CrossRef]
43. Meunier, L.; Aguadé, A.S.; Videau, Y.; Verboux, D.; Fagot-Campagna, A.; Gastaldi-Menager, C.; Amadou, C. Age, Male Gender, and Social Deprivation Are Associated with a Lower Rate of Insulin Pump Therapy Initiation in Adults with Type 1 Diabetes: A Population-Based Study. *Diabetes Technol. Ther.* **2021**, *23*, 8–19. [CrossRef] [PubMed]
44. Kamrath, C.; Tittel, S.R.; Kapellen, T.M.; von dem Berge, T.; Heidtmann, B.; Nagl, K.; Menzel, U.; Pötzsch, S.; Konrad, K.; WHoll, R. Early versus delayed insulin pump therapy in children with newly diagnosed type 1 diabetes: Results from the multicentre, prospective diabetes follow-up DPV registry. *Lancet Child Adolesc. Health* **2021**, *5*, 17–25. [CrossRef]

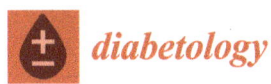

Article
Sex-Gender Differences in Diabetic Retinopathy

Sara Cherchi [1,*], Alfonso Gigante [2], Maria Anna Spanu [3], Pierpaolo Contini [4], Gisella Meloni [5], Maria Antonietta Fois [6], Danila Pistis [2], Rosangela M. Pilosu [4], Alessio Lai [7], Salvatore Ruiu [8], Ilaria Campesi [9] and Giancarlo Tonolo [1,*]

1. SC Diabetologia Aziendale ASSL Olbia, 07026 Olbia, Italy
2. Diabetologia ASSL Nuoro, 08100 Nuoro, Italy; alfonso.gigante@atssardegna.it (A.G.); danila.pistis@atssardegna.it (D.P.)
3. Diabetologia ASSL Sassari, 07100 Sassari, Italy; mariaanna.spanu@atssardegna.it
4. Diabetologia San Giovanni di Dio AOU Cagliari, 09121 Cagliari, Italy; pierpaolocontini@aouca.it (P.C.); rosangelamaria.pilosu@atssardegna.it (R.M.P.)
5. Diabetologia ASSL Lanusei, 08045 Lanusei, Italy; gisella.meloni@atssardegna.it
6. Diabetologia Isili ASSL Cagliari, 09121 Cagliari, Italy; mariaantonietta.fois@atssardegna.it
7. Diabetologia Senorbì ASSL Cagliari, 09121 Cagliari, Italy; alessio.lai@atssardegna.it
8. Poliambulatorio Oculistica ASSL Olbia, 07026 Olbia, Italy; distretto.olbia@atssardegna.it
9. Department Scienze Biomediche, Università degli Studi di Sassari, 07100 Sassari, Italy; ilacampesi79@yahoo.it
* Correspondence: cherchisara@yahoo.it (S.C.); giancarlo.tonolo@atssardegna.it (G.T.)

Received: 30 January 2020; Accepted: 14 April 2020; Published: 20 April 2020

Abstract: Diabetic retinopathy (DR) is one of the main causes of visual loss in individuals aged 20–64 years old. The aim of this study was to investigate, in a multicenter retrospective cross-sectional study, sex-gender difference in DR in a large sample of type 2 diabetic patients (T2DM). 20,611 T2DM regularly attending the units for the last three years were classified as having: (a) No DR (NDR), (b) nonproliferative DR (NPDR), or (c) preproliferative/proliferative DR (PPDR). DR of all grades was present in 4294 T2DM (20.8%), with a significant higher prevalence in men as compared to women (22.0% vs. 19.3% $p < 0.0001$). Among DR patients, both NPDR and PPDR were significantly more prevalent in men vs. women ($p = 0.001$ and $p = 0.0016$, respectively). Women had similar age and BMI, but longer diabetes duration, worse glycemic metabolic control, and more prevalence of hypertension and chronic renal failure (CRF) of any grade vs. men. No significant differences between sexes were evident in term of drug therapy for diabetes and associate pathologies. Conclusions: In this large sample of T2DM, men show higher prevalence of DR vs. women, in spite of less represented risk factors, suggesting that male sex per se might be a risk factor for DR development.

Keywords: diabetes complications; type 2 diabetes; microvascular complications

---

1. Introduction

Diabetic retinopathy (DR) is one of the main causes of visual loss in diabetic subjects of age between 20 and 64 years [1]. Diabetic retinopathy can be classified as nonproliferative (NPDR), usually mild where the walls of the blood vessels in the retina weaken with tiny bulges (microaneurysms) protruding from the vessel walls of the smaller vessels, sometimes leaking fluid and blood into the retina far away from the macula. NPDR can progress to a more severe type, sometimes termed preproliferative, characterized by leaking fluid and/or blood closely to the macula, which is a prelude to the more advanced form of proliferative diabetic retinopathy. In proliferative diabetic retinopathy, damaged blood vessels close off, causing the growth of new, abnormal blood vessels in the retina, and can leak into the clear vitreous, possibly ending in visual loss [1].

Careful control of glycaemia and blood pressure can reduce the risk of developing DR and delay its progression [2]. Higher HBA1c level, diabetes duration, hypertension, and chronic renal failure are globally recognized risk factors for the development of DR [3–6].

Differences between men and women, both in type 1 and type 2 diabetes incidence and in the development of chronic complications, have been reported by several epidemiological studies [7–9]. Controversial results are available in the literature regarding DR and sex-gender differences. Some studies report a higher risk of DR among men [10–14], while others suggest that women might have a higher prevalence of DR than men [15–17]. A clinic-based retrospective longitudinal study with Japanese type 2 diabetes mellitus patients indicated female sex as an independent risk factor for the development of DR, with female sex showing higher prevalence of proliferative DR at baseline [18]. Only a few old reports do not show significant gender difference [19]. Moreover, DR progresses during pregnancy [20,21], suggesting a possible role of sex hormones in retinal damage in diabetes [22,23]. The controversial results on gender differences in DR might be related to ethnic differences, population selection with sometimes mixed T1DM and T2DM subjects or otherwise not well specified, low numbers of observations, and differences in drug treatment for diabetes or associated pathologies between sexes.

As new therapies for diabetic retinopathy are available (from laser-based therapies to vitrectomy and intravitreal corticosteroids, antivascular endothelial growth factors, and more advanced stem cells and ribonucleic acid interference technologies), it becomes demanding to evaluate all the risk factors of DR onset from a gender perspective. Gender is generally considered a social construct that manifests as female in women and male in men, whereas sex is considered the biological aspect of femininity and masculinity. Sex and gender have numerous interactions [24], and sometimes it is difficult to divide sex from gender; thus, it is preferable to adopt "sex-gender" terminology that strongly suggests that the two concepts are jointed. Differences and inequalities in health status often derive from both biological differences and social, cultural, and political arrangements in society. Therefore, we will use this term through this paper.

The aim of this study was to investigate possible sex-gender differences in DR in a large cohort of Sardinian type 2 diabetes (T2DM) patients in a retrospective cross-sectional study.

2. Methods

A multicenter observational retrospective cross-sectional study was carried out on T2DM patients from seven diabetes care units located in different areas of Sardinia: Olbia (OT), Sassari (SS), Nuoro (NU), Lanusei (LA), Isili (IS), Cagliari (CA), and Selargius (SE).

The study was approved by the "Comitato di Bioetica" ATS Sardegna on 27 Jan 2015.

We selected patients with established diagnosis of T2DM regularly attending the Unit from more than three years with at least two coincident eye examination in the period 2016–2018. Diagnosis of type 2 diabetes was done according to the presence of fasting blood glucose more than 126 mg/dL, glycated hemoglobin more than 6.5%, or blood glucose more than 200 mg/dL at 120' of an 75 g Oral Glucose Tolerance test or blood glucose more than 200 mg/dL at any time with symptoms. Out of a total of 29,785 T2DM (16,852 men and 12,933 women), 8242 did not fulfill the enrolment criteria (T2DM diagnosis criteria, irregular attendance to the operative Unit, no coincident eye examination in the period 2016–2018 available) and were excluded. From the remaining 21,543 T2DM patients (12,154 men and 9389 women) enrolled, 932 had maculopathy, and in the remaining 20,611 patients, the prevalence of DR of any grade was 20.8%.

These 20,611 T2DM subjects were divided in two sets: Set 1: patients with HbA1c aggregation data and eye examination (13,267: 7704 men and 5564 women) these patients were enrolled in the OT, SS, and NU diabetes care units; Set 2: patients with only eye examination (7344: 3969 men and 3375 women) these patients were enrolled in the LA, IS, SE, and CA diabetes care units. Set 2 was selected to confirm/deny the results of a different rate of DR between men and women, which was eventually found in set one.

In addition, full clinical data extracted from the clinical database of the Olbia operative unit (OT) were available for 5362 T2DM patients (3003 men and 2359 women). HbA1c, body mass index (BMI), creatinine, urinary albumin excretion rate, total and HDL cholesterol, and triglycerides (TG) were extrapolated from the database, and the mean of the data for any single patient in the last available year was used. Estimated glomerular filtration fraction (eGFR) was calculated with the MDRD equation [25], LDL cholesterol was calculated with the Friedewal formula [(total cholesterol-HDL-Cholesterol)/triglycerides]. Chronic renal failure of any grade was defined from eGFR < 60 mL/min/m^2 in two consecutive occasions at least one month apart, and hypertension as blood pressure > 140/90 mmHg in three different occasions or antihypertensive drug use.

DR was classified after full midriatic eye observation by an ophthalmologists as: (a) no signs of DR (NDR), (b) nonproliferative mild to moderate DR (NPDR), (c) preproliferative/proliferative DR (PPDR), and (d) maculopathy (MAC) [26].

The primary endpoint was the evaluation of sex-gender differences in the different grades of DR, while secondary endpoints included the association between DR and clinical and biochemical parameters in T2DM men and women as well as the sex-gender differences in DR associated diseases and therapies.

Numerical variables were represented as mean ± standard deviation (SD), and categorical variables were presented as frequencies and percentages. Bivariate analysis was performed using Student's *t*-test for continuous variables and chi^2 test for categorical variables. Statistical significance was set at 5% level. A *p*-value of <0.05 was deemed statistically significant.

Logistic regression analysis was performed in the 5362 T2DM patients of the Olbia Unit to identify independent risk factors for diabetic retinopathy using sex as categorical variable and blood pressure, diabetes duration, triglycerides, and HbA1c as continuous variables.

3. Results

All selected patients attended the outpatient clinics regularly without significant differences between males and females. For the flow chart of the study see supplementary material (Figure S1). Nine hundred thirty-two T2DM patients had maculopathy (MAC: 481 men and 451 women) with no significant sex-gender differences. In set 1 (7704 men and 5563 women), DR of any grade was significantly more represented in men (NPDR 16.5% vs. 14.6% *p* = 0.0017 and PPDR 6.5% vs. 5.5% *p* = 0.01), indicating that men having more DR than women (Figure 1).

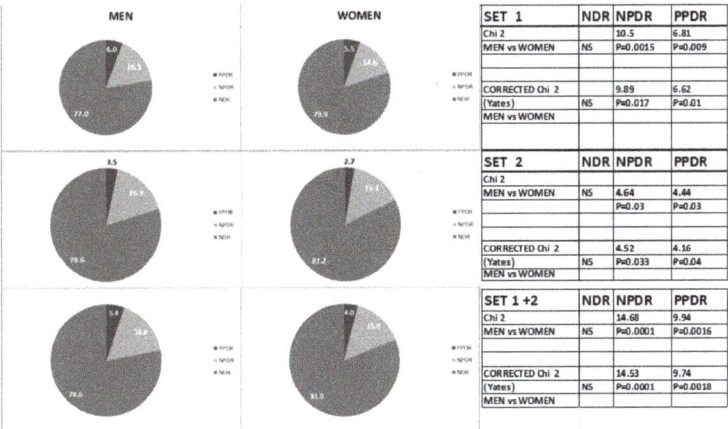

Figure 1. Percentage of diabetic retinopathy (DR) in T2DM patients divided for sex and DR grade [No DR (NDR); Non proliferative DR (NPDR), and pre-proliferative/proliferative DR (PPDR)] in set 1, set 2 and in Set 1+2, respectively. Tables represents the results of Chi 2 analysis.

This data was confirmed in the independent analysis performed in set 2 (3969 men and 3375 women) with a significant prevalence of DR in men (NPDR 16.9% vs. 15.1% $p = 0.03$ and PPDR 3.5% vs. 2.7% $p = 0.04$, Figure 1). When data from set one and two were joined (11,673 men and 8938 women), men confirmed having a significantly higher rate of DR of any grade ($p < 0.0001$) and individually for NPDR ($p = 0.001$) and PPDR $p = 0.0018$) in comparison to women (Figure 1). Since premenopausal women represented 2.6% of the women sample (144/5563 in set 1 and 81/3375 in set 2), no attempt to stratify women in pre/postmenopausal status was made.

Table 1 reports data for T2DM patients of set 1 divided by DR class and HbA1c ≤ 7%, >7% or >8%: women consistently showed higher prevalence of subjects in all classes of DR, with HbA1c over 7% or over 8% being significantly in the NPDR group, indicating generally worse metabolic control in the women group.

Table 1. Diabetic retinopathy grade and HbA1c ≤ 7%, >7%, or HbA1c > 8% of T2DM patients of set 1 (Olbia (OT), Sassari (SS), Nuoro (NU) = 13,267 T2DM) divided by sex (MEN, WOMEN).

	Number	SEX	HbA1c ≤ 7%	HbA1c > 7%	HbA1c > 8%
NRD	5936	MEN	51.9%	48.1%	14.0%
	4443	WOMEN	48.8%	51.2%	14.8%
NPDR	1269	MEN	42.0%	58.0% *	18.8% **
	813	WOMEN	33.9%	66.1% *	25.2% **
PPDR	499	MEN	27.9%	72.1%	29.1%
	307	WOMEN	25.4%	74.6%	29.4%

Chi 2 * $p = 0.006$ ** $p = 0.007$, Corrected Chi2 = (Yates) * $p = 0.0000$, ** $p = 0.0001$. No diabetic retinopathy (NDR) Nonproliferative diabetic retinopathy (NPDR), preproliferative/proliferative diabetic retinopathy (PPDR). Data are reported as %.

Clinical data were available for T2DM patients of OT unit (5362 T2DM patients: men 3003 and women 2359). In this additional subset, men showed higher prevalence of DR as compared to women (NPDR $p = 0.041$, PPDR $p = 0.033$). In these patients, subjects with NPDR and PPDR were older, showed a longer diabetes duration, worse metabolic control, and lower eGFR in comparison to NDR (Table 2).

Table 2. Data from the 5362 T2DM (WOMEN 2359, MEN 3003) of the Olbia operative Unit: Distribution of diabetic retinopathy and clinical parameters divided by sex (MEN, WOMEN) and diabetic retinopathy grade.

		NDR	NPDR	PPDR
Age (years)	MEN	68.1 ± 8.6	74.0 ± 10.2 ⊤	73.1 ± 8.0 ⊤
	WOMEN	68.8 ± 9.0	75.3 ± 9.9 ℂ	73.0 ± 8.1 ℂ
DD (years)	MEN	10.1 ± 5.4	17.0 ± 9.9 ⊤. ***	21 ± 10 ⊤
	WOMEN	10.4 ± 5.4	20.3 ± 10.7 ℂ	22 ± 10 ℂ
BMI (kg/m2)	MEN	29.4 ± 3.7	29.0 ± 6	30.0 ± 5.2
	WOMEN	29.8 ±4.7	31.1 ± 12	31.4 ± 6.8
HbA1c (%)	MEN	6.8 ± 0.9 *	7.3 ± 1.4 ⊤. *	7.8 ± 1.1 ⊤. *
	WOMEN	7.0 ± 0.9	7.5 ± 1.3 ℂ	8.3 ± 1.7 ℂ
Total cholesterol (mg/dL)	MEN	162 ± 27 ***	163 ± 35	156 ± 38
	WOMEN	174 ± 27	168 ± 39	160 ± 39
HDL (mg/dL)	MEN	44 ± 9 ***	45 ± 12 ***	42 ± 9.9 **
	WOMEN	51 ± 10	51 ± 16	49 ± 13
LDL (mg/dL)	MEN	115 ± 62	96 ± 46 ***	100 ± 50
	WOMEN	114 ± 4	110 ± 66	118 ± 42
TG (mg/dL)	MEN	105 ± 32 ***	116 ± 31	90 ± 28
	WOMEN	104 ± 31	116 ± 30	92 ± 38
Creatinine (μmol/L)	MEN	88.0 ± 32.4 ***	96.0 ± 46 ***	103.5 ± 44.9
	WOMEN	74.0 ± 31.0	82. 8 ± 44.1 ℂ	91.8 ± 66.7 ℂ
AER (mg/L)	MEN	32 ± 108 ***	56 ± 159 ⊤. ***	85 ± 178 ⊤. *
	WOMEN	26 ± 94	16 ± 45	45 ± 112
eGFR (mL/min/m2)	MEN	77 ± 29	67 ± 39	62 ± 38 ⊤
	WOMEN	71 ± 26	60 ± 35	54 ± 42 ℂ

No diabetic retinopathy (NDR) Nonproliferative diabetic retinopathy (NPDR), preproliferative/proliferative diabetic retinopathy (PPDR). MEN vs. WOMEN = * $p < 0.05$, ** $p < 0.01$, *** $p < 0.001$; Within MEN vs. NDR = ⊤ $p < 0.001$; Within WOMEN vs. NDR = ℂ $p < 0.01$, ℂ $p < 0.001$.

Women showed significantly higher values, in comparison with men, for diabetes duration ($p < 0.001$ in NPDR), HbA1c ($p < 0.05$ in all classes), HDL-cholesterol ($p < 0.01$ in all classes) and LDL-cholesterol ($p < 0.001$ in NPDR), while BMI, total cholesterol, and TG were similar in men and women in the different groups without significant differences. Creatinine was higher in men, but no differences in calculated eGFR was evident between men and women. In the different classes (NDR, NPDR and PPDR), in both sexes, eGFR decreased constantly while diabetes duration and age increased, again without significant differences between men and women. Albumin excretion rate (AER) was somehow significantly higher in men in all groups.

Finally, associated pathologies were analyzed for T2DM patients of OT unit (Table 3).

Table 3. Data for associated pathologies: Hypertension (HT) and chronic renal failure any grade (CKF) in the 5362 T2DM of the Olbia operative Unit. Distribution of diabetic retinopathy and clinical parameters divided for sex (MEN, WOMEN) and diabetic retinopathy grade.

	NDR MEN = 2331 WOMEN = 1912		NPDR MEN = 504 WOMEN = 344		PPDR MEN = 168 WOMEN = 103	
	HT	CKF	HT	CKF	HT	CKF
MEN %	20.3	6.1	30.3	6.6	14.8	11
WOMEN %	27.3	4.7	33.7	8.9	20.1	22.5
Chi2	$p = 0.0000$	$p = 0.002$	ns	ns	ns	$p = 0.0000$
Corrected Chi2	$p = 0.0000$	$p = 0.002$	ns	ns	ns	$p = 0.0000$

No diabetic retinopathy (NDR) Nonproliferative diabetic retinopathy (NPDR), preproliferative and proliferative diabetic retinopathy (PPDR). Results are given as % of subjects.

Women had more hypertension in all DR classes, being significant in NDR and PPDR. Chronic renal failure (CRF) had a higher prevalence in NDR men in comparison with NDR women, while it was significantly higher in PPDR women than in PPDR men.

No significant difference between men and women were present in drug therapy for diabetes or for antihypertensive drugs or lipid lowering drug use. Among antihypertensive drugs, no significant differences in Angiotensin Converting Enzyme Inhibitors (ACEI) or Angiotensin II Receptor Blockers (ARB) use was present between men and women as well as in the use of statins (Table 4).

Table 4. Drug therapy for diabetes and associated pathologies in the 5362 T2DM patients of Olbia operative unit divided for sex (MEN, WOMEN) and diabetic retinopathy grade.

SEX	MEN	WOMEN
N (%)	3003 (56)	2359 (44)
DIABETES THERAPY (%)		
DIET	6.5	5.8
DIET/OHA	61.9	59.3
OHA + I	12.7	15.2
I	18.9	19.7
OTHER DRUG THERAPY %		
ANTI HYPERTENSIVE	62	59
ACEI/ARB USE	51.8	52.2
LIPID LOWERING	48	48
STATIN USE	94.1	92.5

No diabetic retinopathy (NDR) Nonproliferative diabetic retinopathy (NPDR), preproliferative/proliferative diabetic retinopathy (PPDR). OHA = Oral Antidiabetic Drugs, OHA + I = Oral Antidiabetic Drugs + Insulin, I = Insulin, ACEI/ARB = Converting Enzyme Inhibitors/Angiotensin Receptor Blockers. Data are reported as %. No significant differences between Men and Women.

The logistic regression analysis performed in the Olbia patients indicated sex as the only significant variable.

4. Discussion

DM is associated with an increased risk of cardiovascular mortality, and, in this context, there are evidences highlighting the fact that diabetic women are at a higher risk than their male counterparts, particularly postmenopausal women [27]. While sex-gender differences in macrovascular complications are well established, less is known about microvascular complications in T2DM.

In our population, the prevalence of DR was 20.8%, slightly lower than described in other sets [28–32]. Although our prevalence seems lower than described in other sets, we have to remember that in the other realities, diabetic operative units deal mainly with complicated T2DM patients, while in Sardinia, more than 95% of the diabetic population attend a diabetic operative unit. This data is also important to define a better epidemiologic DR rate among T2DM patients, which in our Sardinian population appears to be approximately 20.8%.

Sex-gender differences in diabetes and in some diabetic complications are well defined, but in DR, these differences are less evident, due to the heterogeneity of the published studies in terms of ethnic origin of the population studied, number of patients analyzed, and selection bias. Male sex is generally, but not always, considered an independent risk factor for DR. Besides what has already been discussed in the introduction, several studies give controversial results on sex-gender differences in diabetic retinopathy. A large-scale study performed in the United States revealed that in diabetic patients over the age of 40 years, men show a 50% higher prevalence of diabetic retinopathy than women [17]. On the other hand, the LALES study [33] showed no statistically significant difference in the incidence of DR between the two sexes. Other studies have also shown this [1,34–37]. The UKPDS 50 study [38] also found no difference in prevalence between the two sexes ($p = 0.67$), with women showing a lower rate of progression of DR than men. In addition, data from a large clinical register in Denmark show no clear sex-gender differences in DR rate, but men have a higher risk for experiencing sight-threatening DR [39].

Male sex seems to be a risk factor for diabetes in adults as well as in juveniles, at least for western countries [40–42], while it is quite the opposite in countries where the population is of non-European origin, in which the prevalence of diabetes seems to be higher in women [43]. Among our patients, women represented 43% of the sample. In some studies that found male sex as a risk factor for DR, men also showed higher HbA1c levels and higher systolic and diastolic blood pressure values than women. Since these are risk factors for progression of DR [44], it could explain the sex-gender difference in the progression rate of DR found in men as an increased presence of additional risk factors for DR. The imbalanced distribution of risk factors among genders could be caused by differences in lifestyle [39], although sex hormones might have a role. DR often progresses during pregnancy, which is associated with higher estrogen and progesterone levels [45,46]. However, it has been demonstrated that women following a tight metabolic control regimen during pregnancy do not show an elevated risk for progression of DR, although the risk often increases again in the postpartum period, since this tight metabolic regimen frequently is no longer followed [45–47].

Mortality and disability after a first vascular event are higher in women, and there are evidences reporting that women receive less medical care regarding cardiovascular complications even in presence of diabetes, or, in any case, reach targets less frequently. From published studies, it appears clear that: (1) women come later and in worse clinical conditions to diagnosis of diabetes, (2) women are more obese at diagnosis and reach guideline target goals for glycated hemoglobin, LDL-cholesterol, or blood pressure control to a much lesser extent [48]; (3) women have a lesser chance of receiving all the diagnostic and therapeutic measures than diabetic men, even if it is well known that mortality after a first cardiovascular event is more elevated in diabetic women [49,50]; (4) finally, some antiaggregating and antihypertensive drugs seem to be less efficacious in diabetic WOMEN, while side effects of some hypoglycemic agents seem to be more frequent, reducing treatment compliance. In a recent ongoing prospective study, the side effects of metformin were shown to have the same incidence in men and women, but with the latter showing greater intensity and duration of these side effects, which affects compliance to drug treatment (preliminary personal observation). Studies focused on sex-gender differences in diabetic microvascular complications are indeed scarcely represented, both at the preclinical and clinical level, mainly due to the well-known limitations of inclusion criteria in trials, but also due to the difficulty of dissecting genetic and environment interactions. Certainly, the lack of capacity to directly target the mechanism initiating the disease, instead of the epiphenomenon, is the cause of the partial failure in the control of diabetic microvascular complication, and this is true in sex-gender oriented medicine as well. Neuroretinal dysfunction can be used to predict the location of future retinopathy up to three years before it manifests, and recently, in adult type 2 diabetic patients, an abnormal local neuroretinal function as been shown in men as compared to women [51]. If confirmed, this might be an alternative explanation for the higher prevalence of diabetic retinopathy in male subjects, in spite of the fact that women had more risk factors for diabetic retinopathy onset and progression.

In this large set of Sardinian T2DM patients, we show that women and men equally receive drug therapy for diabetes and associated pathologies (mainly hypertension and hypercholesterolemia), but women have greater prevalence of hypertension and chronic renal failure and show worse glycemic metabolic control, as is known in the literature [8,9]. The less satisfactory results of drug therapy obtained in women may be related to a different physiological response in the two sexes to the drugs (e.g., the statins), or a difference in adverse drug reactions that result in less compliance to the treatment.

RAAS modulators, mainly ACEI and ARB, may reduce onset and progression of DR in normotensive Type 1 diabetic patients [52,53], and these drugs are able to cause regression of mild DR in normoalbuminuric Type 2 diabetic patients [54]. A recent meta-analysis pointed out that RASS modulators (ACEI more than ARB) might indeed reduce onset and progression of DR in normotensive diabetic patients [55]. In the OT subset of patients, no difference in ACEI/ARB use was evident between men and women.

Finally, the role of sex hormones on retinal disorder must be considered. Recently, the subject has been reviewed [56]. It appears that estrogens, androgens, and progesterone receptors are present throughout the eye and that these steroids are locally produced in ocular tissues. The estrogenic cycle might have a beneficial effect on neuroretinal function, with estrogens, via a vasodilator effect on retinal perfusion, being protective, while testosterone and progesterone, via a vasocostrictive effect, might be a cause of progression. Although interesting, the effect of sex hormones on the retina and their contribution to retinal disorders remain to be proved.

A limitation of this study is that is not a longitudinal study able to detect, in a gender-oriented manner, who might have more rapid progression to DR. A longitudinal prospective study is starting now with these patients and hopefully in the next years we will clarify this aspect.

There are some strengths in this paper: (1) the big sample size of enrolled patients; (2) the multicenter design with the enrollment done in seven different operative units and the replication of the results in two different sets; (3) more than 98% of T2DM patients in Sardinia refer to a diabetes operative unit, resulting in a clear picture of the real prevalence of retinopathy in T2DM patients; and (4) comprehensive data on potential confounders variables in 5362 T2DM patients.

5. Conclusions

In conclusion, in our large sample of T2DM patients, women, although having the same drug treatment as men, showed worse glycemic metabolic control and higher prevalence of hypertension and chronic renal failure, all of which are well-established risk factors for DR, but men showed higher prevalence of DR of any grade, suggesting an independent sex-gender effect. Whether male sex is a cause of diabetic retinopathy development, or female sex is protective, remains to be proven.

Supplementary Materials: The following are available online at http://www.mdpi.com/2673-4540/1/1/s1, Figure S1: Flow chart of the study.

Author Contributions: S.C. and G.T. designed the research; A.G., M.A.S., P.C., G.M., M.A.F., D.P., R.M.P. and A.L. conducted the research; S.C., G.T. and I.C. analyzed the data, S.R. review of doubtful cases of diabetic retinopathy and S.C. wrote the manuscript. G.T. had primary responsibility for the final content. All authors read and approved the final manuscript.

Funding: This research received no external funding.

Acknowledgments: We thank Flavia Franconi for discussion and input given to the realization of this study. S.C. and G.T. are member of the scientific association JANASDIA.

Conflicts of Interest: The authors declare no conflict of interest.

References

1. Zhang, X.; Saaddine, J.B.; Chou, C.F.; Cotch, M.F.; Cheng, Y.J.; Geiss, L.S.; Gregg, E.W.; Albright, A.L.; Klein, B.E.K.; Klein, R. Prevalence of diabetic retinopathy in the United States, 2005–2008. *JAMA* **2010**, *304*, 649–656. [CrossRef] [PubMed]
2. Lachin, J.M.; White, N.H.; Hainsworth, D.P.; Sun, W.; Cleary, P.A.; Nathan, D.M. Effect of intensive diabetes therapy on the progression of diabetic retinopathy in patients with type 1 diabetes: 18 years of follow-up in the DCCT/EDIC. *Diabetes* **2015**, *64*, 631–642. [PubMed]
3. Schanzlin, D.J.; Jay, W.H.; Fritz, K.J.; Tripathi, R.C.; Gonen, B. Hemoglobin A1 and diabetic retinopathy. *Am. J. Ophthalmol.* **1979**, *88*, 1032–1038. [CrossRef]
4. Kaewput, W.; Thongprayoon, C.; Rangsin, R.; Ruangkanchanasetr, P.; Mao, M.A.; Cheungpasitporn, W. Associations of renal function with diabetic retinopathy and visual impairment in type 2 diabetes: A multicenter nationwide cross-sectional study. *World J. Nephrol.* **2019**, *8*, 33–43. [CrossRef] [PubMed]
5. Jenchitr, W.; Samaiporn, S.; Lertmeemongkolchai, P.; Chongwiriyanurak, T.; Anujaree, P.; Chayaboon, D.; Pohikamjorn, A. Prevalence of diabetic retinopathy in relation to duration of diabetes mellitus in community hospitals of Lampang. *J. Med. Assoc. Thai* **2004**, *87*, 1321–1326. [PubMed]
6. Associazione Medici Diabetologi and Società Italiana di Diabetologia (Ed.) *Standard Italiani per la Cura del Diabete Mellito AMD-SID*; Associazione Medici Diabetologi and Società Italiana di Diabetologia: Rome, Italy, 2016; Available online: http://www.siditalia.it/pdf/Standard%20di%20Cura%20AMD%20-%20SID%202018_protetto.pdf (accessed on 27 April 2018).
7. Campesi, I.; Franconi, F.; Seghieri, G.; Meloni, M. Sex-gender-related therapeutic approaches for cardiovascular complications associated with diabetes. *Pharm. Res.* **2017**, *119*, 195–207. [CrossRef]
8. Franconi, F.; Campesi, I.; Occhioni, S.; Tonolo, G. Sex-gender differences in diabetes vascular complications and treatment. *Endocr. Metab. Immune Disord. Drug Targets* **2012**, *12*, 179–196. [CrossRef]
9. Seghieri, G.; Policardo, L.; Anichini, R.; Franconi, F.; Campesi, I.; Cherchi, S.; Tonolo, G. aThe Effect of Sex and Gender on Diabetic Complications. *Curr. Diabetes Rev.* **2016**, *13*, 148–160. [CrossRef]
10. Al-Rubeaan, K.; Abu El-Asrar, A.M.; Youssef, A.M.; Subhani, S.N.; Ahmad, N.A.; Al-Sharqawi, A.H.; Almutlaq, H.M.; David, S.K.; Alnaqeb, D. Diabetic retinopathy and its risk factors in a society with a type 2 diabetes epidemic: A Saudi National Diabetes Registry-based study. *Acta Ophthalmol.* **2015**, *93*, e140–e147. [CrossRef]
11. Pradeepa, R.; Anitha, B.; Mohan, V.; Ganesan, A.; Rema, M. Risk factors for diabetic retinopathy in a South Indian Type 2 diabetic population–the Chennai Urban Rural Epidemiology Study (CURES) Eye Study 4. *Diabet Med.* **2008**, *25*, 536–542. [CrossRef]
12. Rani, P.K.; Raman, R.; Chandrakantan, A.; Pal, S.S.; Perumal, G.M.; Sharma, T. Risk factors for diabetic retinopathy in self-reported rural population with diabetes. *J. Postgrad. Med.* **2009**, *55*, 92–96. [PubMed]
13. Kashani, A.H.; Zimmer-Galler, I.E.; Shah, S.M.; Dustin, L.; Do, D.V.; Eliott, D.; Haller, J.A.; Nguyen, Q.D. Retinal thickness analysis by race, gender, and age using Stratus OCT. *Am. J. Ophthalmol.* **2010**, *149*, 496–502 e1. [CrossRef]
14. Hammes, H.P.; Welp, R.; Kempe, H.P.; Wagner, C.; Siegel, E.; Holl, R.W. Risk Factors for Retinopathy and DME in Type 2 Diabetes-Results from the German/Austrian DPV Database. *PLoS ONE* **2015**, *10*, e0132492. [CrossRef] [PubMed]
15. Constable, I.J.; Knuiman, M.W.; Welborn, T.A.; Cooper, R.L.; Stanton, K.M.; McCann, V.J.; Grose, G.C. Assessing the risk of diabetic retinopathy. *Am. J. Ophthalmol.* **1984**, *97*, 53–61. [CrossRef]
16. West, K.M.; Ahuja, M.M.; Bennett, P.H.; Grab, B.; Grabauskas, V.; Mateo-de-Acosta, O.; Fuller, J.H.; Jarrett, R.J.; Keen, H.; Kosaka, K.; et al. Interrelationships of microangiopathy, plasma glucose and other risk factors in 3583 diabetic patients: A multinational study. *Diabetologia* **1982**, *22*, 412–420. [CrossRef] [PubMed]

17. Deshpande, A.D.; Harris-Hayes, M.; Schootman, M. Epidemiology of diabetes and diabetes-related complications. *Phys. Ther.* **2008**, *88*, 1254–1264. [CrossRef] [PubMed]
18. Kajiwara, A.; Miyagawa, H.; Saruwatari, J.; Kita, A.; Sakata, M.; Kawata, Y.; Oniki, K.; Yoshida, A.; Jinnouchi, H.; Nakagawa, K. Gender differences in the incidence and progression of diabetic retinopathy among Japanese patients with type 2 diabetes mellitus: A clinic-based retrospective longitudinal study. *Diabetes Res. Clin. Pr.* **2014**, *103*, e7–e10. [CrossRef] [PubMed]
19. Pirart, J. Diabetes mellitus and its degenerative complications: A prospective study of 4,400 patients observed between 1947 and 1973 (author's transl). *Diabete Metab* **1977**, *3*, 97–107.
20. Jervell, J.; Moe, N.; Skjaeraasen, J.; Blystad, W.; Egge, K. Diabetes mellitus and pregnancy–management and results at Rikshospitalet, Oslo, 1970–1977. *Diabetologia* **1979**, *16*, 151–155. [CrossRef]
21. Moloney, J.B.; Drury, M.I. The effect of pregnancy on the natural course of diabetic retinopathy. *Am. J. Ophthalmol.* **1982**, *93*, 745–756. [CrossRef]
22. Solomon, S.D.; Chew, E.; Duh, E.J.; Sobrin, L.; Sun, J.K.; VanderBeek, B.L.; Wykoff, C.C.; Gardner, T.W. Diabetic retinopathy: A position statement by the American Diabetes Association. *Diabetes Care* **2017**, *40*, 412–418. [CrossRef] [PubMed]
23. Madendag, Y.; Acmaz, G.; Atas, M.; Sahin, E.; Tayyar, A.T.; Madendag, I.C.; Ozdemir, F.; Senol, V. The effect of oral contraceptive pills on the macula, the retinal nerve fiber layer, and choroidal thickness. *Med. Sci. Monit.* **2015**, *23*, 5657–5661. [CrossRef]
24. Marino, M.; Masella, R.; Bulzomi, P.; Campesi, I.; Malorni, W.; Franconi, F. Nutrition and human health from a sex-gender perspective. *Mol. Asp. Med.* **2011**, *32*, 1–70. [CrossRef] [PubMed]
25. Levey, A.S.; Stevens, L.A.; Schmid, C.H.; Zhang, Y.L.; Castro, A.F., 3rd; Feldman, H.I.; Kusek, J.W.; Eggers, P.W.; van Lente, F.; Greene, T.; et al. A new equation to estimate glomerular filtration rate. *Ann. Intern. Med.* **2009**, *150*, 604–612. [CrossRef]
26. Ellis, D.; Burgess, P.I.; Kayange, P. Management of diabetic retinopathy. *Malawi Med. J.* **2013**, *25*, 116–120.
27. Hu, G. Gender difference in all-cause and cardiovascular mortality related to hyperglycaemia and newly-diagnosed diabetes. *Diabetologia* **2003**, *46*, 608–617. [CrossRef] [PubMed]
28. Yau, J.W.; Rogers, S.L.; Kawasaki, R.; Lamoureux, E.L.; Kowalski, J.W.; Bek, T.; Chen, S.; Dekker, J.M.; Fletcher, A.E.; Grauslund, J.; et al. Global prevalence and major risk factors of diabetic retinopathy. *Diabetes Care* **2012**, *35*, 556–564. [CrossRef]
29. Disoteo, O.; Grimaldi, F.; Papini, E.; Attanasio, R.; Tonutti, L.; Pellegrini, M.A.; Guglielmi, R.; Borretta, G. State-of-the-Art Review on Diabetes Care in Italy. *Ann. Glob. Health* **2015**, *81*, 803–813. [CrossRef]
30. Segato, T.; Midena, E.; Grigoletto, F.; Zucchetto, M.; Fedele, D.; Piermarocchi, S.; Crepaldi, G. The epidemiology and prevalence of diabetic retinopathy in the Veneto region of north east Italy. Veneto Group for Diabetic Retinopathy. *Diabetes Med.* **1991**, *8*, S11–S16. [CrossRef]
31. Porta, M.; Taulaigo, A.V. The changing role of the endocrinologist in the care of patients with diabetic retinopathy. *Endocrine* **2014**, *46*, 199–208. [CrossRef]
32. Cruciani, F.; Abdolrahimzadeh, S.; Vicari, A.; Amore, F.M.; Di Pillo, S.; Mazzeo, L. Causes of blind certification in an Italian province and comparison with other European countries. *Clin. Ter.* **2010**, *161*, e11–e16.
33. Mazhar, K.; Varma, R.; Choudhury, F.; McKean-Cowdin, R.; Shtir, C.J.; Azen, S.P. Severity of diabetic retinopathy and health-related quality of life: The Los Angeles Latino Eye Study. *Ophthalmology* **2011**, *118*, 649–655. [CrossRef]
34. De Block, C.E.; De Leeuw, I.H.; Van Gaal, L.F. Impact of overweight on chronic microvascular complications in type 1 diabetic patients. *Diabetes Care* **2005**, *28*, 1649–1655. [CrossRef]
35. Kostev, K.; Rathmann, W. Diabetic retinopathy at diagnosis of type 2 diabetes in the UK: A database analysis. *Diabetologia* **2013**, *56*, 109–111. [CrossRef]
36. Hammes, H.P.; Kerner, W.; Hofer, S.; Kordonouri, O.; Raile, K.; Holl, R.W. Diabetic retinopathy in type 1 diabetes-a contemporary analysis of 8,784 patients. *Diabetologia* **2011**, *54*, 1977–1984. [CrossRef]
37. Raman, R.; Rani, P.K.; Reddi Rachepalle, S.; Gnanamoorthy, P.; Uthra, S.; Kumaramanickavel, G.; Sharma, T. Prevalence of diabetic retinopathy in India: Sankara Nethralaya Diabetic Retinopathy Epidemiology and Molecular Genetics Study report 2. *Ophthalmology* **2009**, *116*, 311–318. [CrossRef]
38. Stratton, I.M.; Kohner, E.M.; Aldington, S.J.; Turner, R.C.; Holman, R.R.; Manley, S.E.; Matthews, D.R. UKPDS 50: Risk factors for incidence and progression of retinopathy in Type II diabetes over 6 years from diagnosis. *Diabetologia* **2001**, *44*, 156–163. [CrossRef]

39. Mehlsen, J.; Erlandsen, M.; Poulsen, P.L.; Bek, T. Identification of independent risk factors for the development of diabetic retinopathy requiring treatment. *Acta Ophthalmol.* **2011**, *89*, 515–521. [CrossRef]
40. Kaiser, A.; Vollenweider, P.; Waeber, G.; Marques-Vidal, P. Prevalence, awareness and treatment of type 2 diabetes mellitus in Switzerland: The CoLaus study. *Diabet. Med.* **2012**, *29*, 190–197. [CrossRef]
41. Maahs, D.M.; West, N.A.; Lawrence, J.M.; Mayer-Davis, E.J. Epidemiology of type 1 diabetes. *Endocrinol. Metab. Clin. N. Am.* **2010**, *39*, 481–497. [CrossRef]
42. Awa, W.L.; Fach, E.; Krakow, D.; Welp, R.; Kunder, J.; Voll, A.; Zeyfang, A.; Wagner, C.; Schütt, M.; Boehm, B.; et al. Type 2 diabetes from pediatric to geriatric age: Analysis of gender and obesity among 120,183 patients from the German/Austrian DPV database. *Eur. J. Endocrinol.* **2012**, *167*, 245–254. [CrossRef]
43. Cunningham-Myrie, C.; Younger-Coleman, N.; Tulloch-Reid, M.; McFarlane, S.; Francis, D.; Ferguson, T.; Gordonstrachan, G.; Wilks, R. Diabetes mellitus in Jamaica: Sex differences in burden, risk factors, awareness, treatment and control in a developing country. *Trop. Med. Int. Health* **2013**, *18*, 1365–1378. [CrossRef]
44. Matthews, D.R.; Stratton, I.M.; Aldington, S.J.; Holman, R.R.; Kohner, E.M. Risks of progression of retinopathy and vision loss related to tight blood pressure control in type 2 diabetes mellitus: UKPDS 69. *Arch. Ophthalmol.* **2004**, *122*, 1631–1640.
45. Errera, M.H.; Kohly, R.P.; da Cruz, L. Pregnancy-associated retinal diseases and their management. *Surv. Ophthalmol.* **2013**, *58*, 127–142. [CrossRef]
46. Negrato, C.A.; Mattar, R.; Gomes, M.B. Adverse pregnancy outcomes in women with diabetes. *Diabetol. Metab. Syndr.* **2012**, *4*, 41. [CrossRef]
47. Lauszus, F.; Klebe, J.G.; Bek, T. Diabetic retinopathy in pregnancy during tight metabolic control. *Acta Obs. Gynecol. Scand.* **2000**, *79*, 367–370. [CrossRef]
48. Rossi, M.C.; Cristofaro, M.R.; Gentile, S.; Lucisano, G.; Manicardi, V.; Mulas, M.F.; Napoli, A.; Nicolucci, A.; Pellegrini, F.; Suraci, C.; et al. Sex disparities in the quality of diabetes care: Biological and cultural factors may play a different role for different outcomes: A cross-sectional observational study from the AMD Annals initiative. *Diabetes Care* **2013**, *36*, 3162–3168. [CrossRef]
49. Policardo, L.; Seghieri, G.; Francesconi, P.; Anichini, R.; Franconi, F.; Seghieri, C.; del Prato, S. Gender difference in diabetes-associated risk of first-ever and recurrent ischemic stroke. *J. Diabetes Complicat.* **2015**, *29*, 713–717. [CrossRef]
50. Barrett-Connor, E.; Ferrara, A. Isolated postchallenge hyperglycemia and the risk of fatal cardiovascular disease in older women and men. The Rancho Bernardo Study. *Diabetes Care* **1998**, *21*, 1236–1239. [CrossRef]
51. Ozawa, G.Y.; Bearse, M.A., Jr.; Adams, A.J. Male-female differences in diabetic retinopathy? *Curr. Eye Res.* **2015**, *40*, 234–246. [CrossRef]
52. Chaturvedi, N.; Porta, M.; Klein, R.; Orchard, T.; Fuller, J.; Parving, H.H.; Bilous, R.; Sjolie, A.K. Effect of candesartan on prevention (DIRECT-Prevent 1) and progression (DIRECT-Protect 1) of retinopathy in type 1 diabetes: Randomised, placebo-controlled trials. *Lancet* **2008**, *372*, 1394–1402. [CrossRef]
53. Mauer, M.; Zinman, B.; Gardiner, R.; Suissa, S.; Sinaiko, A.; Strand, T.; Drummond, K.; Donnelly, S.; Goodyer, P.; Gubler, M.C.; et al. Renal and retinal effects of enalapril and losartan in type 1 diabetes. *N. Engl. J. Med.* **2009**, *361*, 40–51. [CrossRef] [PubMed]
54. Sjolie, A.K.; Klein, R.; Porta, M.; Orchard, T.; Fuller, J.; Parving, H.H.; Bilous, R.; Chaturvedi, N. Effect of candesartan on progression and regression of retinopathy in type 2 diabetes (DIRECT-Protect 2): A randomised placebo-controlled trial. *Lancet* **2008**, *372*, 1385–1393. [CrossRef]
55. Wang, B.; Wang, F.; Zhang, Y.; Zhao, S.H.; Zhao, W.J.; Yan, S.L.; Wang, Y. Effects of RAS inhibitors on diabetic retinopathy: A systematic review and meta-analysis. *Lancet Diabetes Endocrinol.* **2015**, *3*, 263–274. [CrossRef]
56. Nuzzi, R.; Scalabrin, S.; Becco, A.; Panzica, G. Gonadal Hormones and Retinal Disorders: A Review. *Front. Endocrinol.* **2018**, *9*, 66. [CrossRef]

Publisher's Note: MDPI stays neutral with regard to jurisdictional claims in published maps and institutional affiliations.

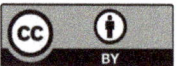

© 2020 by the authors. Licensee MDPI, Basel, Switzerland. This article is an open access article distributed under the terms and conditions of the Creative Commons Attribution (CC BY) license (http://creativecommons.org/licenses/by/4.0/).

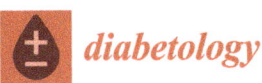

Review

Why We Need Sex-Gender Medicine: The Striking Example of Type 2 Diabetes

Giuseppe Seghieri [1], Flavia Franconi [2] and Ilaria Campesi [2,3,*]

1. Agenzia Regionale Sanità della Toscana, 50141 Firenze, Italy
2. Laboratorio Nazionale di Farmacologia e Medicina di Genere, Istituto Nazionale Biostrutture Biosistemi, 07100 Sassari, Italy
3. Dipartimento di Scienze Biomediche, Università degli Studi di Sassari, 07100 Sassari, Italy
* Correspondence: icampesi@uniss.it

Abstract: Type 2 diabetes mellitus is a widespread and a chronic disease associated with micro- and macrovascular complications and is a well-established risk factor for cardiovascular disease, which are among the most important causes of death in diabetic patients. This disease is strongly affected by sex and gender: sex-gender differences have been reported to affect diabetes epidemiology and risk factors, as well as cardiovascular complications associated with diabetes. This suggests the need for different therapeutic approaches for the management of diabetes-associated complications in men and women. In this review, we describe the known sex-gender differences in diabetic men and women and discuss the therapeutic approaches for their management. The data reported in this review show that a sex-gender approach in medicine is mandatory to maximize the scientific rigor and value of the research. Sex-gender studies need interdisciplinarity and intersectionality aimed at offering the most appropriate care to each person.

Keywords: sex-gender differences; type 2 diabetes mellitus; therapy

1. Introduction

Over the past 20–30 years, research has shown, from single cells to multiple complex biological systems, that biological sex and gender differences are numerous and involve all branches of the biomedical sciences. According to the Council of Europe [1], the term sex regards *"the different biological and physiological characteristics of males and females, such as reproductive organs, chromosomes or hormones"*, whereas gender regards *"the socially constructed characteristics of women and men—such as norms, roles, and relationships of and between groups of women and men"*. Nowadays it is clear that sex and gender interact forming Gordian node [2,3]; thus, it is very difficult to separate them [2–4].

It is important to recognize that sex differences apply to all vertebrates and humans and that sexual dimorphism varies in the species and strains of animals. Sex should, in fact, be considered in all cell studies, as it is now evident that primary cells other than males and females behave differently [5–11]. In diabetes research, as an example, it is very difficult to find an animal model suitable for studying gender differences in the pathology and its complications as different animal models show sexually dimorphic diabetic phenotypes [12].

Moreover, sex-gender differences are highly influenced by age: they, in fact, begin in the uterus. Fetal programming includes also a set of epigenetic changes in response to various environmental stimuli that can affect life and the health of the child even in adulthood [13–16], a phenomenon that was well known by diabetologists because David J Bakers hypothesized that chronic, degenerative conditions of adult health, such as cardiovascular diseases and type 2 diabetes, may be triggered by in utero events [17].

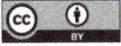

The lack of attention to the sex-gender variable is also found in some clinical studies: the erroneous assumption that men and women are equal has led to the underrepresentation of women in clinical studies or to considering the differences between men and women as normal [18]. A major reason for this shortcoming is that the overall gender-stratified sample size is often too small to produce valid results. Furthermore, despite well-recognized sex and gender differences in disease management, most management guidelines are not sex-gender specific [2,19,20].

In this context, it is important to stress that the pharmacological response is multifactorial and depends not only on the drug but also on patient-related factors, such as genetic and epigenetic factors, age, body composition and metabolism, use of concomitant drugs (including oral contraceptives), and exposure to environmental factors, as well as to socio-cultural factors [11,20–23]. All of this has a strong impact on pharmacokinetics and pharmacodynamics and on the onset of adverse drug reactions, which are more reported by women. They also take more drugs and botanical remedies and experience more interactions with an increased risk of adverse drug reactions [19,24–27].

An interesting and significant example of how sex-gender can influence pathophysiology and therapeutic response is provided by type 2 diabetes [4,28–31].

2. Type 2 Diabetes: A Sex-Gender Disease

Diabetes is one of the most common diseases, with a continuous worldwide rise in its incidence [32]. The toll paid by people with diabetes is the associated huge burden of cardiovascular diseases including coronary artery disease, ischemic stroke, or heart failure; they are going to suffer throughout their life with a reduced quality of life as well as a reduced life expectancy. In this context, an aspect that is emerging with ever greater clarity is that both the pathogenesis of diabetes as well as its cardiovascular complications are significantly sex-gender oriented. Sex, in fact, plays a significant role in determining the risk of developing diabetes, especially type 2 diabetes mellitus, which represents about 90% of all cases of diabetes. First, according to most epidemiological surveys, men are more at risk of diabetes, as compared to women, at least excluding the older strata of the population, where the women seem to be more represented [33]. A lot of evidence has been accrued, during the last decade, suggesting that the metabolic regulation of carbohydrates and lipids is different in women as compared to men [34]. Overall, the female sex is characterized by features that have a protective role against the development of diabetes such as reduced visceral disposition of adiposity, higher total body insulin sensitivity, and greater non-esterified fatty acids oxidation after exercise, with the only exception of the finding that women present greater plasma glucose value after 2-hr- oral glucose tolerance test (OGTT) [4,35]. It is reported that the one shield which protects women against metabolic derangements predisposing them to diabetes, as well as protecting them against its cardiovascular complications, is represented by the exposure to estrogens [36–39]. Estrogens in animal models impressively reduce whole-body adiposity, increase insulin sensitivity and improve overall glucose tolerance [40,41]. This protective action of estrogens, however, is lost with menopause [42], and due to this event, from this date females are being exposed to risk factors for cardiovascular diseases, including diabetes, even more than men.

Numerous studies have investigated the potential mechanisms that may underpin the sex-gender differences in type 2 diabetes mellitus [43–48]. Glycated hemoglobin (HbA1c) is more strongly associated with fasting plasma glucose in women than in men, and age, waist circumference, body max index, systolic and diastolic blood pressure, triglyceride levels, total cholesterol, low density lipoprotein, high density lipoprotein, fasting insulin, and proinsulin levels all predict type 2 diabetes mellitus better in women [45,48].

The impaired fasting glucose/impaired glucose tolerance occurs in a more severe endothelial dysfunction in women than men, including changes in markers of endothelial function (E-selectin and soluble intercellular adhesion molecule). In addition, fibrinolysis (plasminogen activator inhibitor-1) is more abnormal in premenopausal women with type 2 diabetes than their male counterparts [43,44,49]. Moreover, hyperglycemia induces oxidative stress and upregulation of pro-inflammatory factors, promoting a vascular dysfunction [50]. Oxidative stress induces insulin resistance by altering the insulin-signaling pathway and the levels of adipokines nuclear factor kappa-B, tumor necrosis factor α, interleukin 1β plasma endotoxin, and toll-like receptor 4 are increased [50–53].

Metabolic pathways involved in the pathogenesis of diabetes seem to be, therefore, in part, sex determined; however, in this sex dimorphism, even if the effect of estrogens is well delineated, the additional role of other determinants, such as sex chromosomes, gut microbiome, prenatal conditioning events or sex-related epigenetic modifications, cannot be ruled out being the object of ongoing research [54–57].

3. Sex-Gender Differences in Diabetic Complications

As testified by metanalytical studies regarding large populations, women with diabetes have a significantly higher risk of coronary heart disease, stroke, ischemic stroke, or vascular dementia than men [4,54], with the only exclusion being peripheral arterial diseases [58]. All this means that diabetes is associated with a greater adjusted relative risk of cardiovascular events, especially coronary heart diseases and ischemic stroke in women (by ~40%) as compared to men [59,60]. Further proof of concept for this greater diabetes-driven facility of women comes from the recent finding that after hospitalization for diabetic foot, a diabetes complication overwhelmingly associated with male sex, women are more at risk of cardiovascular events such as ischemic stroke or myocardial infarction [61,62]. As compared to people without diabetes, moreover, women are more exposed not only to all complications of diabetes but also to other risk factors for cardiovascular diseases such as obesity, smoking, hypertension, or dyslipidemia. All this is of great importance since all these risk factors are frequently combined, all or in part, in the same woman with diabetes. In addition, interestingly, at diagnosis of diabetes women are on average more obese and have a higher number of either traditional or novel risk factors not at target, as compared to men [63–65]. In conclusion, the burden of diabetes and its macrovascular complications, as well as the relative greater impact of all risk factors for atherosclerosis, is greater among women, being only partly counterbalanced by a lesser absolute risk of diabetes or cardiovascular events, when compared to men [66]. Furthermore, a lot of effort has been made over time to shed light on the role of sex in female disadvantage given to diabetes. In this context, interestingly, recent studies have demonstrated that any causal effect of genetic liability to type 2 diabetes on the risk of coronary heart disease is not stronger for women than men [67], while the impairment in the metabolic control of diabetes, as expressed by each one unit increase in glycated hemoglobin, impacts to the same extent in men and women [68]. Sex-gender aspects, however, cannot be ruled out to explain this greater diabetes-associated risk among women. Inequalities in the treatment of diabetes and of associated vascular risk factors leading to a lesser percentage of women who reach the optimal target after treatment of diabetes [69] or differences in socioeconomic status, mainly disadvantaging women, may be additionally considered causes to explain the reason of this gender-oriented gap. In conclusion, women are more susceptible to cardiovascular complications of diabetes than men are, even if practically this is mitigated by a lesser absolute risk of both diabetes and atherosclerotic events among women. Sex biological, hormonal, and genetic differences associated with gender aspects such as inequalities in treatment or differences in socioeconomic status between men and women may explain and further modulate the extent of this gap. The main lesson for health caregivers is to tailor primary and secondary interventions in people with diabetes, keeping in mind the existence of such sex-gender differences in susceptibility to its vascular complications.

4. Microvascular Complications

The sex-gender impact of diabetes on microvascular complications is much less defined, as compared to what is evidenced for macrovascular complications. Regarding retinopathy, both in type 1 and in type 2 diabetes, its severity, as well as the evolution over time, seems worse among males [70–72]. Studies concerning sex- gender differences in incidence or severity of diabetic nephropathy are more uncertain, with some suggesting men as more affected by renal complications, while others suggest that women are more predisposed to a worse prognosis for end-stage renal disease [73–75]. In this regard, it is interesting to note that women with type 2 diabetes are at greater risk of non-albuminuric renal failure, presumably due to this type of renal damage apparently being most associated with cardiovascular events [76]. There are, however, studies that do not find sex-gender differences in both the incidence and time course of diabetic nephropathy. Regarding diabetic neuropathy, both peripheral sensory-motor and autonomic diabetic neuropathy have been found to be more prevalent in men, even if the reports are conflicting [77–82], due also to the non-standardized methodology in the diagnosis of neuropathy for epidemiological purposes. Finally, it should be emphasized that no clear pathophysiological aspects have been identified to explain the sex-gender-related differences in diabetic microangiopathy, not unlike those suggested for macrovascular complications.

5. Drug Response

Until now the sex and gender influences on drug response have been neglected and the "one size fits all" model is still predominant both in research and in daily clinical practice [2,21,83]. Relevantly, the clinical trials of new antidiabetic drugs enrolled only 20–40% of women [18], and often, some of them have no statistical power to verify whether sex-gender may be related to response differences [84]. The low participation of women leads to reduced appropriateness in women because data are accumulating, pointing out the sex and gender differences in drug prescribing, the pharmacokinetics, the pharmacodynamics, and the efficacy and safety profile of multiple combinations of drugs [18,21].

Concerning diabetes, it should be noted that in diabetic individuals the pharmacokinetics and pharmacodynamics change. In particular, changes in blood flow in subcutaneous adipose tissue and muscle, gastric mobility, and acidity may altogether affect the absorption of drugs [18]. Type 2 diabetes mellitus-induced effects on oral absorption may prevail in women [21]. The gastroenteric diabetic alterations in fact can vary the ionization of weak acids and bases, therefore, changing absorption, as occurs with glipizide [85]. It should be considered, moreover, that healthy women have longer gastrointestinal emptying times and higher gastric pH than men [21]. The sex and gender differences observed in healthy individuals in subcutaneous adipose tissues and skeletal muscle (more fat and less muscle in women) together with blood flow variations could lead to altered subcutaneous and intramuscular absorption of insulin in a sex-specific way [85]. The non-enzymatic glycation of protein may involve drug-metabolizing enzymes altering biotransformation and drug transporters involved in drug elimination. Notably, alterations in pharmacokinetics are drug specific [18]. The obesity present in many diabetic individuals may participate in pharmacokinetic variation observed in diabetics [85]. The effect of diabetes on pharmacodynamics is less known but it cannot be underestimated that type 2 diabetes mellitus alters ions channels [86] increasing the risk of arrhythmias including the prolonging of the QT interval [87], which is longer in women than in men, and being a woman is a risk factor for iatrogenic QT long syndrome. Several recent reviews have brilliantly and exhaustively reported sex and gender differences in pharmacokinetics, pharmacodynamics, and safety profiles available for the different antidiabetics drug classes [18,24], which are summarized in Table 1.

Treatments with new synthetic antidiabetic drugs, namely, sodium-glucose-cotransporter-2 (SGLT2) inhibitors and glucagon-like peptide-1 receptor (GLP-1R) agonists, decrease ischemic events and atherosclerotic cardiovascular disease [84,88]. SGLT2 inhibitors also have cardio-renal benefits even in non-diabetic patients. They reduce hospitalizations and mortality for patients with heart failure with reduced ejection fraction and prevention of progression of chronic kidney disease. However, trials with GLP-1R agonists for cardiovascular risk assessment enrolled only a few women (ranging from 30% with albiglutide (HARMONY) to 46% with dulaglutide (REWIND)) [88]. Trials with SGLT2 inhibitors enrolled even fewer women (ranging from 29% empagliflozin (EMPA-REG-OUTCOME) to 37% with dapagliflozin (Declare-TIMI-58)) [88]. The number of women is still low in the second-generation trials. The absence of women in clinical trials leads to the lack of sex-gender-specific reporting rates. With SGLT2 inhibitors, urinary tract/genital infection dominated in women, while a gastrointestinal drugs effect prevailed in women treated with GLP-1R agonists [29]. In view of sex-gender differences that significantly impact pharmacokinetics and pharmacodynamics [21], research devoted to finding sex-gender differences in drug response is urgent. Still, it is also urgent to identify sex-gender differences, including the higher reporting rates of adverse events in women [3] which will impact pharmacovigilance results.

Table 1. Some sex-gender differences in antidiabetic drugs.

Drug	Differences	References
Insulin	fertile women require higher dose	[24,89,90]
	higher risk of hypoglycaemia in women	[91]
Biguanides	higher reduction in HbA1c in men	[92]
	higher lactic acidosis in women	[93]
	higher treatment failure in women	[94]
Sulfonyureas	higher exposure in women	[95]
	higher weight loss in women	[92]
	lower end-stage kidney disease in men	[96]
Thiazolidinediones	higher exposure to pioglitazone in women	[95]
	higher risk of bone fractures in women	[97,98]
GLP-1R agonists	higher prescription in young women	[84]
	better glycaemic control in men	[84,99]
	higher weight loss in women	[99]
	higher gastrointestinal adverse effects in women	[99]
Alpha glucosidase inhibitors	more effective in older and non-obese women	[100]
	higher gastrointestinal adverse effects in men	[101]
SGLT2 inhibitors	better response in men	[102]
	higher urinary infections in women	[103,104]
	higher ketoacidosis in women	[105,106]
	higher Fournier gangrene in men	[107]

6. Conclusions

The data reported in this review show that a sex-gender approach in medicine is mandatory. To maximize the scientific rigor and value of the research, it is mandatory to include sex and gender in both pre-clinical and clinical research, to ensure health equity and to ameliorate the health and well-being of all citizens. Therefore, sex-gender studies need interdisciplinarity and intersectionality aimed at offering the most appropriate care to each person. Gender biases could be avoided by implementing greater scientific rigor of research, from preclinical to clinical practice, by making a concerted effort to ensure that sex-gender-specific analyses are included, to ensure health equity and appropriateness.

Funding: This research received no external funding.

Conflicts of Interest: The authors declare no conflict of interest.

References

1. Council of Europe Sex and Gender. Available online: https://www.coe.int/en/web/gender-matters/sex-and-gender (accessed on 23 April 2022).
2. Franconi, F.; Campesi, I.; Colombo, D.; Antonini, P. Sex-gender variable: Methodological recommendations for increasing scientific value of clinical studies. *Cells* **2019**, *8*, 476. [CrossRef] [PubMed]
3. Campesi, I.; Montella, A.; Seghieri, G.; Franconi, F. The person's care requires a sex and gender approach. *J. Clin. Med.* **2021**, *10*, 4770. [CrossRef] [PubMed]

4. Seghieri, G.; Policardo, L.; Anichini, R.; Franconi, F.; Campesi, I.; Cherchi, S.; Tonolo, G. The Effect of Sex and Gender on Diabetic Complications. *Curr. Diabetes Rev.* **2017**, *13*, 148–160. [CrossRef]
5. Campesi, I.; Capobianco, G.; Dessole, S.; Occhioni, S.; Montella, A.; Franconi, F. Estrogenic compounds have divergent effects on human endothelial progenitor cell migration according to sex of the donor. *J. Vasc. Res.* **2015**, *52*, 273–278. [CrossRef] [PubMed]
6. Campesi, I.; Marino, M.; Montella, A.; Pais, S.; Franconi, F. Sex differences in estrogen receptor α and β levels and activation status in LPS-stimulated human macrophages. *J. Cell Physiol.* **2017**, *232*, 340–345. [CrossRef]
7. Ruggieri, A.; Gambardella, L.; Maselli, A.; Vona, R.; Anticoli, S.; Panusa, A.; Malorni, W.; Matarrese, P. Statin-induced impairment of monocyte migration is gender-related. *J. Cell Physiol.* **2014**, *229*, 1990–1998. [CrossRef]
8. Straface, E.; Vona, R.; Gambardella, L.; Ascione, B.; Marino, M.; Bulzomi, P.; Canu, S.; Coinu, R.; Rosano, G.; Malorni, W.; et al. Cell sex determines anoikis resistance in vascular smooth muscle cells. *FEBS Lett.* **2009**, *583*, 3448–3454. [CrossRef] [PubMed]
9. Lloret, A.; Badia, M.C.; Mora, N.J.; Ortega, A.; Pallardo, F.V.; Alonso, M.D.; Atamna, H.; Vina, J. Gender and age-dependent differences in the mitochondrial apoptogenic pathway in Alzheimer's disease. *Free Radic. Biol. Med.* **2008**, *44*, 2019–2025. [CrossRef] [PubMed]
10. Du, L.; Hickey, R.W.; Bayir, H.; Watkins, S.C.; Tyurin, V.A.; Guo, F.; Kochanek, P.M.; Jenkins, L.W.; Ren, J.; Gibson, G.; et al. Starving neurons show sex difference in autophagy. *J. Biol. Chem.* **2009**, *284*, 2383–2396. [CrossRef]
11. Campesi, I.; Sanna, M.; Zinellu, A.; Carru, C.; Rubattu, L.; Bulzomi, P.; Seghieri, G.; Tonolo, G.; Palermo, M.; Rosano, G.; et al. Oral contraceptives modify DNA methylation and monocyte-derived macrophage function. *Biol. Sex Differ.* **2012**, *3*, 4. [CrossRef]
12. Franconi, F.; Seghieri, G.; Canu, S.; Straface, E.; Campesi, I.; Malorni, W. Are the available experimental models of type 2 diabetes appropriate for a gender perspective? *Pharmacol. Res.* **2008**, *57*, 6–18. [CrossRef] [PubMed]
13. Caterino, M.; Ruoppolo, M.; Costanzo, M.; Albano, L.; Crisci, D.; Sotgiu, G.; Saderi, L.; Montella, A.; Franconi, F.; Campesi, I. Sex Affects Human Premature Neonates' Blood Metabolome According to Gestational Age, Parenteral Nutrition, and Caffeine Treatment. *Metabolites* **2021**, *11*, 158. [CrossRef]
14. Addis, R.; Campesi, I.; Fois, M.; Capobianco, G.; Dessole, S.; Fenu, G.; Montella, A.; Cattaneo, M.G.; Vicentini, L.M.; Franconi, F. Human umbilical endothelial cells (HUVECs) have a sex: Characterisation of the phenotype of male and female cells. *Biol. Sex Differ.* **2014**, *5*, 18. [CrossRef] [PubMed]
15. Grigore, D.; Ojeda, N.B.; Alexander, B.T. Sex differences in the fetal programming of hypertension. *Gend. Med.* **2008**, *5*, S121–S132. [CrossRef]
16. Barker, D.J. Intrauterine programming of adult disease. *Mol. Med. Today* **1995**, *1*, 418–423. [CrossRef]
17. Barker, D.J.P.; Osmond, C.; Winter, P.D.; Margetts, B.; Simmonds, S.J. Weight in infancy and death from ischaemic heart disease. *Lancet* **1989**, *2*, 577–580. [CrossRef]
18. Campesi, I.; Seghieri, G.; Franconi, F. Type 2 diabetic women are not small type 2 diabetic men: Sex-and-gender differences in antidiabetic drugs. *Curr. Opin. Pharmacol.* **2021**, *60*, 40–45. [CrossRef]
19. Campesi, I.; Racagni, G.; Franconi, F. Just a reflection: Does drug repurposing perpetuate sex-gender bias in the safety profile? *Pharmaceuticals* **2021**, *14*, 730. [CrossRef]
20. Ventura-Clapier, R.; Dworatzek, E.; Seeland, U.; Kararigas, G.; Arnal, J.F.; Brunelleschi, S.; Carpenter, T.C.; Erdmann, J.; Franconi, F.; Giannetta, E.; et al. Sex in basic research: Concepts in the cardiovascular field. *Cardiovasc. Res.* **2017**, *113*, 711–724. [CrossRef]
21. Mauvais-Jarvis, F.; Berthold, H.K.; Campesi, I.; Carrero, J.J.; Dakal, S.; Franconi, F.; Gouni-Berthold, I.; Heiman, M.L.; Kautzky-Willer, A.; Klein, S.L.; et al. Sex- and gender-based pharmacological response to drugs. *Pharmacol. Rev.* **2021**, *73*, 730–762. [CrossRef]
22. Campesi, I.; Romani, A.; Franconi, F. The sex-gender effects in the road to tailored botanicals. *Nutrients* **2019**, *11*, 1637. [CrossRef]
23. Campesi, I.; Marino, M.; Cipolletti, M.; Romani, A.; Franconi, F. Put "gender glasses" on the effects of phenolic compounds on cardiovascular function and diseases. *Eur. J. Nutr.* **2018**, *57*, 2677–2691. [CrossRef] [PubMed]
24. Franconi, F.; Campesi, I. Sex and gender influences on pharmacological response: An overview. *Expert Rev. Clin. Pharmacol.* **2014**, *7*, 469–485. [CrossRef] [PubMed]
25. Regitz-Zagrosek, V.; Oertelt-Prigione, S.; Prescott, E.; Franconi, F.; Gerdts, E.; Foryst-Ludwig, A.; Maas, A.H.; Kautzky-Willer, A.; Knappe-Wegner, D.; Kintscher, U.; et al. Gender in cardiovascular diseases: Impact on clinical manifestations, management, and outcomes. *Eur. Heart. J.* **2016**, *37*, 24–34. [PubMed]
26. Anderson, G.D. Sex and racial differences in pharmacological response: Where is the evidence? Pharmacogenetics, pharmacokinetics, and pharmacodynamics. *J. Womens Health* **2005**, *14*, 19–29. [CrossRef]
27. Soldin, O.P.; Mattison, D.R. Sex differences in pharmacokinetics and pharmacodynamics. *Clin. Pharmacokinet.* **2009**, *48*, 143–157. [CrossRef]
28. Stock, S.A.; Stollenwerk, B.; Redaelli, M.; Civello, D.; Lauterbach, K.W. Sex differences in treatment patterns of six chronic diseases: An analysis from the German statutory health insurance. *J. Womens Health* **2008**, *17*, 343–354. [CrossRef]
29. Joung, K.I.; Jung, G.W.; Park, H.H.; Lee, H.; Park, S.H.; Shin, J.Y. Gender differences in adverse event reports associated with antidiabetic drugs. *Sci. Rep.* **2020**, *10*, 17545. [CrossRef]
30. Franconi, F.; Campesi, I.; Occhioni, S.; Tonolo, G. Sex-gender differences in diabetes vascular complications and treatment. *Endocr. Metab. Immune Disord. Drug Targets* **2012**, *12*, 179–196. [CrossRef]
31. Campesi, I.; Franconi, F.; Seghieri, G.; Meloni, M. Sex-gender-related therapeutic approaches for cardiovascular complications associated with diabetes. *Pharmacol. Res.* **2017**, *119*, 195–207. [CrossRef]

32. Saeedi, P.; Petersohn, I.; Salpea, P.; Malanda, B.; Karuranga, S.; Unwin, N.; Colagiuri, S.; Guariguata, L.; Motala, A.A.; Ogurtsova, K.; et al. Global and regional diabetes prevalence estimates for 2019 and projections for 2030 and 2045: Results from the International Diabetes Federation Diabetes Atlas, 9th edition. *Diabetes Res. Clin. Pract.* **2019**, *157*, 107843. [CrossRef] [PubMed]
33. American Diabetes Association. Classification and diagnosis of diabetes: Standards of medical care in diabetes-2018. *Diabetes Care* **2018**, *41*, S13–S27. [CrossRef]
34. Walden, C.E.; Knopp, R.H.; Wahl, P.W.; Beach, K.W.; Strandness, E. Sex differences in the effect of diabetes mellitus on lipoprotein triglyceride and cholesterol concentrations. *N. Engl. J. Med.* **1984**, *311*, 953–959. [CrossRef] [PubMed]
35. Anderwald, C.; Gastaldelli, A.; Tura, A.; Krebs, M.; Promintzer-Schifferl, M.; Kautzky-Willer, A.; Stadler, M.; DeFronzo, R.A.; Pacini, G.; Bischof, M.G. Mechanism and effects of glucose absorption during an oral glucose tolerance test among females and males. *J. Clin. Endocrinol. Metab.* **2011**, *96*, 515–524. [CrossRef] [PubMed]
36. Kannel, W.B.; Hjortland, M.C.; McNamara, P.; Gordon, T. Menopause and risk of cardiovascular disease: The Framingham study. *Ann. Intern. Med.* **1976**, *85*, 447–452. [CrossRef]
37. Hulley, S.; Grady, D.; Bush, T.; Furberg, C.; Herrington, D.; Riggs, B.; Vittinghoff, E. Randomized trial of estrogen plus progestin for secondary prevention of coronary heart disease in postmenopausal women. Heart and Estrogen/progestin Replacement Study (HERS) Research Group. *JAMA* **1998**, *280*, 605–613. [CrossRef]
38. Rossouw, J.E.; Prentice, R.L.; Manson, J.E.; Wu, L.; Barad, D.; Barnabei, V.M.; Ko, M.; Lacroix, A.Z.; Margolis, K.L.; Stefanick, M.L. Postmenopausal hormone therapy and risk of cardiovascular disease by age and years since menopause. *JAMA* **2007**, *297*, 1465–1477. [CrossRef]
39. Manson, J.E.; Allison, M.A.; Rossouw, J.E.; Carr, J.J.; Langer, R.D.; Hsia, J.; Kuller, L.H.; Cochrane, B.B.; Hunt, J.R.; Ludlam, S.E.; et al. Estrogen therapy and coronary-artery calcification. *N. Engl. J. Med.* **2007**, *356*, 2591–2602. [CrossRef]
40. González-Granillo, M.; Savva, C.; Li, X.; Ghosh Laskar, M.; Angelin, B.; Gustafsson, J.Å.; Korach-André, M. Selective estrogen receptor (ER)β activation provokes a redistribution of fat mass and modifies hepatic triglyceride composition in obese male mice. *Mol. Cell. Endocrinol.* **2020**, *502*, 110672. [CrossRef]
41. Barros, R.P.A.; Gustafsson, J.Å. Estrogen receptors and the metabolic network. *Cell Metab.* **2011**, *14*, 289–299. [CrossRef]
42. Policardo, L.; Seghieri, G.; Francesconi, P.; Anichini, R.; Franconi, F.; Del Prato, S. Gender difference in diabetes related excess risk of cardiovascular events: When does the "risk window" open? *J. Diabetes Complicat.* **2017**, *31*, 74–79. [CrossRef] [PubMed]
43. Donahue, R.P.; Rejman, K.; Rafalson, L.B.; Dmochowski, J.; Stranges, S.; Trevisan, M. Sex differences in endothelial function markers before conversion to pre-diabetes: Does the clock start ticking earlier among women? The Western New York Study. *Diabetes Care* **2007**, *30*, 354–359. [CrossRef]
44. Vanhoutte, P.M. Endothelial dysfunction: The first step toward coronary arteriosclerosis. *Circ. J.* **2009**, *73*, 595–601. [CrossRef] [PubMed]
45. Li, T.; Quan, H.; Zhang, H.; Lin, L.; Lin, L.; Ou, Q.; Chen, K. Type 2 diabetes is more predictable in women than men by multiple anthropometric and biochemical measures. *Sci. Rep.* **2021**, *11*, 1–10. [CrossRef]
46. Peters, S.A.E.; Huxley, R.R.; Sattar, N.; Woodward, M. Sex differences in the excess risk of cardiovascular diseases associated with type 2 diabetes: Potential explanations and clinical implications. *Curr. Cardiovasc. Risk Rep.* **2015**, *9*, 1–7. [CrossRef] [PubMed]
47. Peters, S.A.E.; Huxley, R.R.; Woodward, M. Diabetes as a risk factor for stroke in women compared with men: A systematic review and meta-analysis of 64 cohorts, including 775,385 individuals and 12,539 strokes. *Lancet* **2014**, *383*, 1973–1980. [CrossRef]
48. Giustino, G.; Redfors, B.; Mehran, R.; Kirtane, A.J.; Baber, U.; Généreux, P.; Witzenbichler, B.; Neumann, F.J.; Weisz, G.; Maehara, A.; et al. Sex differences in the effect of diabetes mellitus on platelet reactivity and coronary thrombosis: From the Assessment of Dual Antiplatelet Therapy with Drug-Eluting Stents (ADAPT-DES) study. *Int. J. Cardiol.* **2017**, *246*, 20–25. [CrossRef]
49. Huebschmann, A.G.; Huxley, R.R.; Kohrt, W.M.; Zeitler, P.; Regensteiner, J.G.; Reusch, J.E.B. Sex differences in the burden of type 2 diabetes and cardiovascular risk across the life course. *Diabetologia* **2019**, *62*, 1761–1772. [CrossRef]
50. Contreras-Zentella, M.L.; Hernández-Muñoz, R. Possible gender influence in the mechanisms underlying the oxidative stress, inflammatory response, and the metabolic alterations in patients with obesity and/or type 2 diabetes. *Antioxidants* **2021**, *10*, 1729. [CrossRef]
51. Aljada, A.; Mohanty, P.; Ghanim, H.; Abdo, T.; Tripathy, D.; Chaudhuri, A.; Dandona, P. Increase in intranuclear nuclear factor kappaB and decrease in inhibitor kappaB in mononuclear cells after a mixed meal: Evidence for a proinflammatory effect. *Am. J. Clin. Nutr.* **2004**, *79*, 682–690. [CrossRef]
52. Houstis, N.; Rosen, E.D.; Lander, E.S. Reactive oxygen species have a causal role in multiple forms of insulin resistance. *Nature* **2006**, *440*, 944–948. [CrossRef] [PubMed]
53. Evans, J.L.; Maddux, B.A.; Goldfine, I.D. The molecular basis for oxidative stress-induced insulin resistance. *Antioxid. Redox. Signal.* **2005**, *7*, 1040–1052. [CrossRef] [PubMed]
54. Kautzky-Willer, A.; Harreiter, J.; Pacini, G. Sex and gender differences in risk, pathophysiology and complications of type 2 diabetes mellitus. *Endocr. Rev.* **2016**, *37*, 278–316. [CrossRef]
55. Zore, T.; Palafox, M.; Reue, K. Sex differences in obesity, lipid metabolism, and inflammation-A role for the sex chromosomes? *Mol. Metab.* **2018**, *15*, 35–44. [CrossRef]
56. Weger, B.D.; Gobet, C.; Yeung, J.; Martin, E.; Jimenez, S.; Betrisey, B.; Foata, F.; Berger, B.; Balvay, A.; Foussier, A.; et al. The mouse microbiome is required for sex-specific diurnal rhythms of gene expression and metabolism. *Cell Metab.* **2019**, *29*, 362–382.e8. [CrossRef] [PubMed]

57. Dearden, L.; Bouret, S.G.; Ozanne, S.E. Sex and gender differences in developmental programming of metabolism. *Mol. Metab.* **2018**, *15*, 8–19. [CrossRef]
58. Chase-Vilchez, A.Z.; Chan, I.H.Y.; Peters, S.A.E.; Woodward, M. Diabetes as a risk factor for incident peripheral arterial disease in women compared to men: A systematic review and meta-analysis. *Cardiovasc. Diabetol.* **2020**, *19*, 151. [CrossRef]
59. Maric-Bilkan, C. Sex differences in micro- and macro-vascular complications of diabetes mellitus. *Clin. Sci.* **2017**, *131*, 833–846. [CrossRef]
60. Peters, S.A.E.; Huxley, R.R.; Woodward, M. Diabetes as risk factor for incident coronary heart disease in women compared with men: A systematic review and meta-analysis of 64 cohorts including 858,507 individuals and 28,203 coronary events. *Diabetologia* **2014**, *57*, 1542–1551. [CrossRef]
61. Seghieri, G.; Policardo, L.; Gualdani, E.; Anichini, R.; Francesconi, P. Gender difference in the risk for cardiovascular events or mortality of patients with diabetic foot syndrome. *Acta Diabetol.* **2019**, *56*, 561–567. [CrossRef]
62. Seghieri, G.; De Bellis, A.; Seghieri, M.; Gualdani, E.; Policardo, L.; Franconi, F.; Francesconi, P. Gender difference in the risk of adverse outcomes after diabetic foot disease: A mini-review. *Curr. Diabetes Rev.* **2021**, *17*, 207–213. [CrossRef] [PubMed]
63. Schroeder, E.B.; Bayliss, E.A.; Daugherty, S.L.; Steiner, J.F. Gender differences in cardiovascular risk factors in incident diabetes. *Womens Health Issues* **2014**, *24*, e61–e68. [CrossRef] [PubMed]
64. Wannamethee, S.G.; Papacosta, O.; Lawlor, D.A.; Whincup, P.H.; Lowe, G.D.; Ebrahim, S.; Sattar, N. Do women exhibit greater differences in established and novel risk factors between diabetes and non-diabetes than men? The British Regional Heart Study and British Women's Heart Health Study. *Diabetologia* **2012**, *55*, 80–87. [CrossRef] [PubMed]
65. Millett, E.R.C.; Peters, S.A.E.; Woodward, M. Sex differences in risk factors for myocardial infarction: Cohort study of UK Biobank participants. *BMJ* **2018**, *363*, k4247. [CrossRef]
66. Peters, S.A.E.; Woodward, M. Sex, gender, and precision medicine. *JAMA Intern. Med.* **2020**, *180*, 1128–1129. [CrossRef] [PubMed]
67. Peters, T.M.; Holmes, M.V.; Brent Richards, J.; Palmer, T.; Forgetta, V.; Lindgren, C.M.; Asselbergs, F.W.; Nelson, C.P.; Samani, N.J.; McCarthy, M.I.; et al. Sex differences in the risk of coronary heart disease associated with type 2 diabetes: A mendelian randomization analysis. *Diabetes Care* **2021**, *44*, 556–562. [CrossRef]
68. de Jong, M.; Woodward, M.; Peters, S.A.E. Diabetes, glycated hemoglobin, and the risk of myocardial infarction in women and men: A prospective cohort study of the uk biobank. *Diabetes Care* **2020**, *43*, 2050–2059. [CrossRef]
69. Rossi, M.C.; Cristofaro, M.R.; Gentile, S.; Lucisano, G.; Manicardi, V.; Mulas, M.F.; Napoli, A.; Nicolucci, A.; Pellegrini, F.; Suraci, C.; et al. Sex disparities in the quality of diabetes care: Biological and cultural factors may play a different role for different outcomes: A cross-sectional observational study from the amd annals initiative. *Diabetes Care* **2013**, *36*, 3162–3168. [CrossRef]
70. Harjutsalo, V.; Maric, C.; Forsblom, C.; Thorn, L.; Wadén, J.; Groop, P.H. Sex-related differences in the long-term risk of microvascular complications by age at onset of type 1 diabetes. *Diabetologia* **2011**, *54*, 1992–1999. [CrossRef]
71. Looker, H.C.; Nyangoma, S.O.; Cromie, D.; Olson, J.A.; Leese, G.P.; Black, M.; Doig, J.; Lee, N.; Lindsay, R.S.; McKnight, J.A.; et al. Diabetic retinopathy at diagnosis of type 2 diabetes in Scotland. *Diabetologia* **2012**, *55*, 2335–2342. [CrossRef]
72. Kostev, K.; Rathmann, W. Diabetic retinopathy at diagnosis of type 2 diabetes in the UK: A database analysis. *Diabetologia* **2013**, *56*, 109–111. [CrossRef] [PubMed]
73. Sibley, S.D.; Thomas, W.; De Boer, I.; Brunzell, J.D.; Steffes, M.W. Gender and elevated albumin excretion in the Diabetes Control and Complications Trial/Epidemiology of Diabetes Interventions and Complications (DCCT/EDIC) cohort: Role of central obesity. *Am. J. Kidney Dis.* **2006**, *47*, 223–232. [CrossRef] [PubMed]
74. Jacobsen, P.; Rossing, K.; Tarnow, L.; Rossing, P.; Mallet, C.; Poirier, O.; Cambien, F.; Parving, H.H. Progression of diabetic nephropathy in normotensive type 1 diabetic patients. *Kidney Int.* **1999**, *71*, S101–S105. [CrossRef] [PubMed]
75. Cherney, D.Z.I.; Sochett, E.B.; Miller, J.A. Gender differences in renal responses to hyperglycemia and angiotensin-converting enzyme inhibition in diabetes. *Kidney Int.* **2005**, *68*, 1722–1728. [CrossRef] [PubMed]
76. Penno, G.; Solini, A.; Bonora, E.; Fondelli, C.; Orsi, E.; Zerbini, G.; Trevisan, R.; Vedovato, M.; Gruden, G.; Cavalot, F.; et al. Clinical significance of nonalbuminuric renal impairment in type 2 diabetes. *J. Hypertens.* **2011**, *29*, 1802–1809. [CrossRef]
77. Dyck, P.J.; Kratz, K.M.; Karnes, J.L.; Litchy, W.J.; Klein, R.; Pach, J.M.; Wilson, D.M.; O'Brien, P.C.; Melton, L.J. The prevalence by staged severity of various types of diabetic neuropathy, retinopathy, and nephropathy in a population-based cohort: The Rochester Diabetic Neuropathy Study. *Neurology* **1993**, *43*, 817–824. [CrossRef]
78. Albers, J.W.; Brown, M.B.; Sima, A.A.F.; Greene, D.A. Nerve conduction measures in mild diabetic neuropathy in the Early Diabetes Intervention Trial: The effects of age, sex, type of diabetes, disease duration, and anthropometric factors. Tolrestat Study Group for the Early Diabetes Intervention Trial. *Neurology* **1996**, *46*, 85–91. [CrossRef]
79. Booya, F.; Bandarian, F.; Larijani, B.; Pajouhi, M.; Nooraei, M.; Lotfi, J. Potential risk factors for diabetic neuropathy: A case control study. *BMC Neurol.* **2005**, *5*, 1–5. [CrossRef]
80. Brown, M.J.; Bird, S.J.; Watling, S.; Kaleta, H.; Hayes, L.; Eckert, S.; Foyt, H.L. Natural progression of diabetic peripheral neuropathy in the Zenarestat study population. *Diabetes Care* **2004**, *27*, 1153–1159. [CrossRef]
81. Dyck, P.J.; Litchy, W.J.; Hokanson, J.L.; Low, J.L.; O'Brien, P.C. Variables influencing neuropathic endpoints: The Rochester Diabetic Neuropathy Study of Healthy Subjects. *Neurology* **1995**, *45*, 1115–1121. [CrossRef]
82. Pop-Busui, R.; Lu, J.; Lopes, N.; Jones, T.L.Z. Prevalence of diabetic peripheral neuropathy and relation to glycemic control therapies at baseline in the BARI 2D cohort. *J. Peripher. Nerv. Syst.* **2009**, *14*, 1–13. [CrossRef] [PubMed]

83. Stillhart, C.; Vučićević, K.; Augustijns, P.; Basit, A.W.; Batchelor, H.; Flanagan, T.R.; Gesquiere, I.; Greupink, R.; Keszthelyi, D.; Koskinen, M.; et al. Impact of gastrointestinal physiology on drug absorption in special populations—An UNGAP review. *Eur. J. Pharm. Sci.* **2020**, *147*, 105280. [CrossRef] [PubMed]
84. Raparelli, V.; Elharram, M.; Moura, C.S.; Abrahamowicz, M.; Bernatsky, S.; Behlouli, H.; Pilote, L. Sex differences in cardiovascular effectiveness of newer glucose-lowering drugs added to metformin in type 2 diabetes mellitus. *J. Am. Heart Assoc.* **2020**, *9*, e012940. [CrossRef]
85. Dostalek, M.; Akhlaghi, F.; Puzanovova, M. Effect of diabetes mellitus on pharmacokinetic and pharmacodynamic properties of drugs. *Clin. Pharmacokinet.* **2012**, *51*, 481–499. [CrossRef]
86. Ozturk, N.; Uslu, S.; Ozdemir, S. Diabetes-induced changes in cardiac voltage-gated ion channels. *World J. Diabetes* **2021**, *12*, 1–18. [CrossRef]
87. Vasheghani, M.; Sarvghadi, F.; Beyranvand, M.R.; Emami, H. The relationship between QT interval indices with cardiac autonomic neuropathy in diabetic patients: A case control study. *Diabetol. Metab. Syndr.* **2020**, *12*, 102. [CrossRef] [PubMed]
88. Ferro, E.G.; Elshazly, M.B.; Bhatt, D.L. New antidiabetes medications and their cardiovascular and renal benefits. *Cardiol. Clin.* **2021**, *39*, 335–351. [CrossRef]
89. Trout, K.K.; Rickels, M.R.; Schutta, M.H.; Petrova, M.; Freeman, E.W.; Tkacs, N.C.; Teff, K.L. Menstrual cycle effects on insulin sensitivity in women with type 1 diabetes: A pilot study. *Diabetes Technol. Ther.* **2007**, *9*, 176–182. [CrossRef]
90. McGill, J.B.; Vlajnic, A.; Knutsen, P.G.; Recklein, C.; Rimler, M.; Fisher, S.J. Effect of gender on treatment outcomes in type 2 diabetes mellitus. *Diabetes Res Clin Pract.* **2013**, *102*, 167–174. [CrossRef]
91. Jovanovic, L. Sex differences in insulin dose and postprandial glucose as BMI increases in patients with type 2 diabetes. *Diabetes Care* **2009**, *32*, e148. [CrossRef]
92. Schutt, M.; Zimmermann, A.; Hood, R.; Hummel, M.; Seufert, J.; Siegel, E.; Tytko, A.; Holl, R.W. Gender-specific Effects of Treatment with Lifestyle, Metformin or Sulfonylurea on Glycemic Control and Body Weight: A German Multicenter Analysis on 9 108 Patients. *Exp. Clin. Endocrinol. Diabetes* **2015**, *123*, 622–626. [CrossRef] [PubMed]
93. Li, Q.; Liu, F.; Tang, J.L.; Zheng, T.S.; Lu, J.X.; Lu, H.J.; Jia, W.P. The gender difference of plasma lactate levels and the influence of metformin in type 2 diabetes patients. *Chin. J. Endocrinol. Metab.* **2010**, *26*, 372–376.
94. Mamza, J.; Mehta, R.; Donnelly, R.; Idris, I. Important differences in the durability of glycaemic response among second-line treatment options when added to metformin in type 2 diabetes: A retrospective cohort study. *Ann. Med.* **2016**, *48*, 224–234. [CrossRef] [PubMed]
95. Karim, A.; Zhao, Z.; Slater, M.; Bradford, D.; Schuster, J.; Laurent, A. Replicate study design in bioequivalency assessment, pros and cons: Bioavailabilities of the antidiabetic drugs pioglitazone and glimepiride present in a fixed-dose combination formulation. *J. Clin. Pharmacol.* **2007**, *47*, 806–816. [CrossRef]
96. Wong, M.G.; Perkovic, V.; Chalmers, J.; Woodward, M.; Li, Q.; Cooper, M.E.; Hamet, P.; Harrap, S.; Heller, S.; Macmahon, S.; et al. Long-term Benefits of Intensive Glucose Control for Preventing End-Stage Kidney Disease: ADVANCE-ON. *Diabetes Care* **2016**, *39*, 694–700. [CrossRef]
97. Kahn, S.E.; Haffner, S.M.; Viberti, G.; Herman, W.H.; Lachin, J.M.; Kravitz, B.G.; Yu, D.; Paul, G.; Holman, R.R.; Zinman, B. Rosiglitazone decreases C-reactive protein to a greater extent relative to glyburide and metformin over 4 years despite greater weight gain: Observations from a Diabetes Outcome Progression Trial (ADOPT). *Diabetes Care* **2010**, *33*, 177–183. [CrossRef]
98. Aubert, R.E.; Herrera, V.; Chen, W.; Haffner, S.M.; Pendergrass, M. Rosiglitazone and pioglitazone increase fracture risk in women and men with type 2 diabetes. *Diabetes Obes. Metab.* **2010**, *12*, 716–721. [CrossRef]
99. Anichini, R.; Cosimi, S.; Di Carlo, A.; Orsini, P.; De Bellis, A.; Seghieri, G.; Franconi, F.; Baccetti, F. Gender difference in response predictors after 1-year exenatide therapy twice daily in type 2 diabetic patients: A real world experience. *Diabetes Metab. Syndr. Obes.* **2013**, *6*, 123–129.
100. West, D.S.; Elaine Prewitt, T.; Bursac, Z.; Felix, H.C. Weight loss of black, white, and Hispanic men and women in the Diabetes Prevention Program. *Obesity* **2008**, *16*, 1413–1420. [CrossRef]
101. Chiasson, J.L.; Josse, R.G.; Gomis, R.; Hanefeld, M.; Karasik, A.; Laakso, M. Acarbose for prevention of type 2 diabetes mellitus: The STOP-NIDDM randomised trial. *Lancet* **2002**, *359*, 2072–2077. [CrossRef]
102. Han, E.; Kim, A.; Lee, S.J.; Kim, J.Y.; Kim, J.H.; Lee, W.J.; Lee, B.W. Characteristics of dapagliflozin responders: A longitudinal, prospective, nationwide dapagliflozin surveillance study in Korea. *Diabetes Ther.* **2018**, *9*, 1689–1701. [CrossRef] [PubMed]
103. Dave, C.V.; Schneeweiss, S.; Kim, D.; Fralick, M.; Tong, A.; Patorno, E. Sodium-glucose cotransporter-2 inhibitors and the risk for severe urinary tract infections: A population-based cohort study. *Ann. Intern. Med.* **2019**, *171*, 248–256. [CrossRef] [PubMed]
104. FDA SGLT2 Inhibitors: Drug Safety Communication—Labels to Include Warnings about Too Much Acid in the Blood and Serious Urinary Tract Infections. Available online: https://www.fda.gov/safety/medwatch/safetyinformation/safetyalertsforhumanmedicalproducts/ucm475553.htm (accessed on 6 June 2022).
105. Blau, J.E.; Tella, S.H.; Taylor, S.I.; Rother, K.I. Ketoacidosis associated with SGLT2 inhibitor treatment: Analysis of FAERS data. *Diabetes. Metab. Res. Rev.* **2017**, *33*, e2924. [CrossRef]

106. Palmer, B.F.; Clegg, D.J. Euglycemic ketoacidosis as a complication of SGLT2 inhibitor therapy. *Clin. J. Am. Soc. Nephrol.* **2021**, *16*, 1284–1291. [CrossRef]
107. Bersoff-Matcha, S.J.; Chamberlain, C.; Cao, C.; Kortepeter, C.; Chong, W.H. Fournier gangrene associated with sodium-glucose cotransporter-2 inhibitors: A review of spontaneous postmarketing cases. *Ann. Intern. Med.* **2019**, *170*, 764–769. [CrossRef] [PubMed]

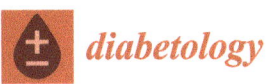

Review

Gender Difference in Type 1 Diabetes: An Underevaluated Dimension of the Disease †

Patrizio Tatti * and Singh Pavandeep

Istituto I.N.I.–Via S. Anna SNC, Grottaferrata, 00046 Roma, Italy; pavanmaan97@gmail.com
* Correspondence: info@patriziotatti.it
† Proceedings from "Gender differences in diabetes" held in Olbia, 4–5 December 2020.

Abstract: Gender difference in all fields of medicine and biology has recently become a topic of great interest. At present, most studies report gender differences in their secondary analysis; however, this information receives scant attention from clinicians, and is often overwhelmed by press trumpeting the overall main positive results. Furthermore, and more importantly, any statistical evaluation of results obtained without specific and careful planning in the study for the topic of research is probably worthless. There are few studies in animals, but these are not typically useful because of the different biology, pharmacodynamics and pharmacokinetics compared to humans. Type 1 diabetes is a disease where gender difference can be easily evaluated. Irrespective of the cause of the loss of pancreatic beta-cell function, the common denominators of all forms of type 1 diabetes are the absence of circulating insulin and a reduction in peripheral insulin sensitivity leading to exogenous injections being required. Consequently, exogenous insulin infusion, with any of the widely used research tools, such as the insulin–glucose clamp, can be easily used to evaluate gender difference. Female patients with type 1 diabetes have many factors that impact glucose level. For example, the hormones that drive the ovulatory/menstrual cycle and the connected change at the time of the menopause have a role on insulin action; thus, one should expect great research emphasis on this. On the contrary, there is a dearth of data available on this topic, and no pump producer has created a gender-specific insulin infusion profile. Patients are usually approached on the basis of their diagnosis. This review is intended to focus on personalized treatment, more specifically on gender, according to the modern way of thinking.

Keywords: gender; diabetes; type 1

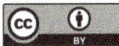

1. Introduction

Type 1 diabetes has many different genetic and environmental causes, and a common pathophysiological ground represented by the almost total or total absence of insulin. Hyperglycemia is the cause of complications in almost all the organs of the body. The appearance, degree, and location of these complications may depend on a number of conditions. Among them are the degree of blood sugar control, the duration of the disease, the age of the patient, the type of insulin used for replacement, the number of injections, the spectrum of residual endogenous insulin secretion, the sensitivity of the peripheral tissue to the insult, the blood glucose swings (glucose variability), and not least the sexual and genetic environment and hormonal patterns. Among these conditions, sex is the simplest to control, although there are not many studies that account for this variable.

Males and females were not created equal. Gender differences are much deeper than the reproductive/sexual dimorphism, and span most of the organs.

Unfortunately, for whatever reason, these differences have been too easily dismissed in medicine and in the socio/economic environment.

We know that the differences involve physiology and also pharmacokinetics and pharmacodynamics. This mini review deals with the gender differences in type I diabetes. It is clear that biological differences play a role, but where, when and how is not clear.

2. Incidence

The incidence of type 1 diabetes varies across latitude, race, and economic conditions. A study in Sweden spanning from 1983 to 2002 found an annual incidence rate of 16.4/100,000 for males and 8.9/100,000 for females [1]. The differences decreased slowly with age, but the prevalence remained higher in men with an overall male/female ratio of 1.8. Notably, temporal trends and seasonal patterns (higher in January–March and lower in May–July) were the same in both sexes, thus pointing the focus to gender rather than exposure to environmental factors.

Another study [2] found an increased risk of T1DM (type 1 diabetes mellitus) in boys with neonatal infections (OR = 2.42, (CI 1.14–5.15) $p = 0.02$) and a decreased risk in girls with neonatal infections (OR = 0.4 (CIU 0.12–1.38) $p = 0.15$). This difference remained unaltered after removing the confounders. Diabetes is a T-cell-mediated autoimmune disease, so the difference may reside in gender-linked susceptibility and response to infections. Many papers have demonstrated sexual dimorphism in the immune cell count and activity between males and females, likely dependent on the sex hormones.

Although the point has been dissected according to age and other characteristics, at present there is no unifying view of the gender gap in type 1 diabetes. A study in Germany dealing with self-assessed adherence to prescriptions reported that poor glycemic control was found in 19% of men and in 18% of women [3].

Contrary to other organ-specific autoimmune disorders, T1DM does not show a female prevalence, with a limited roughly 45% figure [4]. However, the matter is more complicated than this. The populations with the highest prevalence of T1DM show male excess; the reverse is true for populations with low prevalence of the disease. Unfortunately the diagnosis of type 1 diabetes is not always so lear-cut. Type 1 diabetes is a distinctive disease only in children, where it can be diagnosed with utmost confidence. The appearance in these subjects is abrupt and noteworthy. Type 1 DM appears also in advanced age, over 40 years, but the disease often goes undiagnosed and confused with insulin-treated type 2 DM (type 2 diabetes mellitus). In these subjects, the HLA (human leukocyte antigen) type, insulin deficiency and insulin autoantibody changes are less evident than in children [5], or may be absent [6]. Accordingly, it is difficult to draw firm conclusions from studies in this population.

Accordingly, a careful review of prevalence identified a slight excess of males in European countries and a female prevalence in populations of Asian and African origin [7].

When we restrict the observations to those under 15 years of age, we find that in populations with an incidence rate of T1DM over 23/100,000 there is male preponderance, while the reverse is true for those populations with an incidence rate under 4.5/100,000. Another unexpected finding is that in those patients with no islet antibodies there is a strict male predominance [8]. It is difficult to draw firm conclusions from these partially conflicting data.

3. Clinical Aspects

Another study from Edinburgh with no clear-cut age limit reported that women were more likely to seek medical help and feel symptoms. This review indicates that male diabetics are observed to be living more effectively with diabetes, with lesser depression and anxiety and more energy and better wellbeing [9], although diabetic men with advanced disease may experience the phenomenon of erectile dysfunction, which causes serious depression and the tendency to abandon the cure. A similar sex dysfunction with vaginal dryness probably occurs in women, but this has not been investigated in depth. Furthermore, the more sophisticated sex–arousal mechanism of the female body, with relevant psychic influences, makes the topic more complicated.

Another study found that girls may be more likely to hide non-adherence to the prescription of insulin, and consequently may have feelings of guilt and self-blame [10]. This may be in part to do with the phenomenon known as "cheating", which means that girls and young women know that hyperglycemia in diabetes induces the loss of weight, so they voluntarily reduce the insulin dose, even more so in these times of social media exposure where models of fitness and beauty are inspiring the youth.

There are very few data available on insulin action on each sex in type 1 diabetes. We can deduce some useful information to shed light on Type 1 diabetes from the data of men and women patients with type 2 diabetes. We think that some information obtained from a large number of men and women with type 2 diabetes, which is a much more metabolically complex disease, can partially be used to understand the gender differences in Type 1: (i) women appeared to be more sensitive to insulin in regard to glucose metabolism (both in the liver and in muscle); (ii) there were no differences in insulin action on lipolysis in men and women; (iii) the data available on the regulation of triglyceride and protein metabolism by insulin in men and women were too scarce to draw firm conclusions; (iv) there might be differences in the insulin-sensitizing effects of exercise and weight loss in men and women [11].

Furthermore the presence of type 1 diabetes is no guarantee against the appearance of insulin resistance in those affected. Insulin resistance in type 1 can be induced by an increased fat tissue mass due to over-treatment with insulin. Thus, some of the metabolic defects in insulin-resistant type 2 diabetics may also be present in type 1. The role of insulin has been traditionally studied in the context of glucose metabolism. However, insulin also plays a role in the inhibition of adipose tissue lipolysis and fatty acid release into the blood stream [12], regulates hepatic lipid metabolism [13], and inhibits protein breakdown [14]. In addition, insulin action and insulin resistance are not the same in any organ of the body, and we only know a little part of this [15]. It is evident that studying these differences in the intact human body is quite difficult at present, and more so in men and women separately. We know that fasting plasma glucose and glucose production and disposal are apparently not different between sexes [16], although in some studies women exhibited a greater and more prolonged suppression of endogenous glucose production rates than men [17]. This observation, if confirmed, may have great relevance in the management of insulin-induced hypoglycemia. Estrogens that are prevalent in the first part of the menstrual cycle have divergent effects on insulin action, that overall seem to be positive by increasing insulin action on peripheral tissue. Greater rates of glucose disposal during the follicular compared to the luteal phase of the menstrual cycle have been observed during a hyperglycemic (blood glucose > 200 mg/dL) hyperinsulinemic clamp [18]. Progesterone, on the other hand, seems to interfere negatively with insulin action, thus apparently increasing the need for injected insulin in type 1 DM [19].

Other hormones also play a role in this gender difference. Treatment with testosterone reduces insulin-mediated glucose disposal in women [20] and hyperandrogenemia might be the major culprit for insulin resistance in women with polycystic ovary syndrome.

It may seem absurd, but, to our knowledge, no infusion profile that accounts for these subtle cyclic changes in women on CSII (continuous subcutaneous insulin infusion) has been put forward.

There are no clear differences between men and women in terms of insulin action on lipolysis [21], although this should have been viewed in the context of different muscle mass. Finally, overall available data confirm that the response of adipose tissue lipolysis to insulin appears to be the same in the two sexes.

There may be differences in the regulation of plasma triglyceride concentration and protein metabolism by insulin and in changes in insulin action in response to hormonal stimuli. Women appear to be more sensitive to the suppression of VLDL (very-low-density lipoproteins) by insulin [22].

The available results about muscle protein synthesis raise perplexity because, ironically, the papers that do find differences report a greater rate of muscle protein synthesis in women than in men [23]. This was not anticipated because of the well-established anabolic effects of testosterone. Clearly a lot more work must be completed in this field. Some recent data show that the interest to close this gender gap is increasing. This is absolutely necessary because the menstrual cycle with its hormone-driven swings imposes a serious challenge on women, who also have to struggle with subtle disturbing symptoms.

A study at the Mount Sinai Hospital on 16 menstruating women on an insulin-sensor-controlled automated pump, showed that the TIR (time in range) could be improved to 69% in the menstrual phase, 67% during the luteal phase, and 69% during the rest of the cycle. This may affect the lives of women at the fertile age that usually strive to cope with a high blood sugar level during their menstrual cycle. This is just a starting point, but with improved attention to the phenomenon, it is likely that the companies producing these pumps will come out with an algorithm able to create a personalized insulin delivery profile.

4. Conclusions

The gender gap in type 1 diabetes is far from closed. At present, we are still without a clear picture of the biology of blood glucose control in males versus females. In the case of females, we do not know enough about what happens at different ages—prepubertal, post-pubertal reproductive, and after the menopause—and what drives any change. This information is probably relevant to achieve an effective cure for patients with diabetes mellitus. We have known for a long time that the net effect of insulin on the body is the result of pharmacodynamics (effect of insulin on the body) and pharmacokinetics (effect of the body on insulin). So far, we know more on pharmacodynamics, but very little on pharmacokinetics, especially in women. We need to shed light on this to achieve any effective cure.

In conclusion, we have no firm data on gender difference in type 1 diabetes mellitus. Males appear to be more frequently affected by the disease, although this may vary in different populations, and females appear to show higher sensitivity to insulin. This aspect may be of relevance in insulin treatment and in cases of emergency treatment for hypoglycemia. Accordingly, treatment with male hormones appears to increase insulin resistance in women, and this hormonal effect may explain the lower insulin sensitivity in men. Hopefully, future studies will help to tailor a better insulin treatment in both sexes.

5. Patients

This section is not mandatory but may be added if there are patients resulting from the work reported in this manuscript.

Funding: This research received no external funding.

Conflicts of Interest: The author declares no conflict of interest.

References

1. Östman, J.; Lönnberg, G.; Arnqvist, H.J.; Blohme, G.; Bolinder, J.; Schnell, A.E.; Eriksson, J.W.; Gudbjörnsdottir, S.; Sundkvist, G.; Nyström, L. Gender differences and temporal variation in the incidence of type 1 diabetes: Results of 8012 cases in the nationwide Diabetes Incidence Study in Sweden 1983–2002. *J. Intern. Med.* **2008**, *263*, 386–394. [CrossRef] [PubMed]
2. Svensson, J.; Carstensen, B.; Mortensen, H.B.; Borch-Johnsen, K. Gender-associated differences in Type 1 diabetes risk factors? *Diabetologia* **2003**, *46*, 442–443. [CrossRef] [PubMed]
3. Jacqueline, A. Bartlett, Immune Function in healthy Inner-City Children. *Clin. Diagn. Lab. Immunol.* **2001**, *8*, 740–746.
4. McKnight, J.A.; Wild, S.H.; Lamb, M.J.; Cooper, M.N.; Jones, T.W.; Davis, E.A.; Hofer, S.; Fritsch, M.; Schober, E.; Svensson, J.; et al. Glycemic control of type 1 diabetes in clinical practice early in the 21th century. An international comparison. *Diabetic Med.* **2015**, *32*, 1036–1050. [CrossRef]
5. Beeson, P.B. Age and sex association of 40 autoimmune diseases. *Am. J. Med.* **1994**, *96*, 457–462. [CrossRef]
6. Karjalainen, J.; Salmela, P.; Ilonen, J.; Surcel, H.M.; Knip, M. A comparison of childhood and adult Diabetes Mellitus. *NEJM* **1989**, *320*, 881–886. [CrossRef] [PubMed]
7. Wilson, R.M.; Van der Minne, P.; Deverill, I.; Heller, S.R.; Gelsthorpe, K.; Reeves, W.G.; Tattersall, R.B. Insulin dependence: Problems with the classification of 100 consecutive patients. *Dabetic Med.* **1985**, *2*, 167–172. [CrossRef]
8. Karvonen, M.; Pitkäniemi, M.; Pitkäniemi, J.; Kohtamäki, K.; Tajima, N.; Tuomilehto, J. Sex difference in the prevalence of insulin-dependent Diabetes Mellitus. *Diab. Met. Rev.* **1997**, *13*, 275–291. [CrossRef]

9. Weets, I.; Van Der Auwera, B.; Schuit, F.; Du Caju, M.; Decochez, K.; Coeckelberghs, M.; De Leeuw, I.; Keymeulen, B.; Mathieu, C.; Rottiers, R.; et al. Male to female excess in diabetes presenting after the age of 15 years. *Diabetologia* **1999**, *40*, 40–47.
10. Siddiqui, M.A.; Khan, M.F.; Carline, T.E. Gender differences in living with diabetes mellitus. *Mater. Socio-Med.* **2013**, *25*, 140–142. [CrossRef]
11. Raum, E.; Krämer, H.U.; Rüter, G.; Rothenbacher, D.; Rosemann, T.; Szecsenyi, J.; Brenner, H. Medication non adherence and poor glycemic control in patients with type 2 diabetes. *Diabetes Res. Clin. Pract.* **2012**, *97*, 377–384. [CrossRef] [PubMed]
12. Williams, C. Adolescence and the management of diabetes. *J. Adv. Nurs.* **1999**, *30*, 21–36. [CrossRef] [PubMed]
13. Magkos, F.; Wang, X.; Mittendorfer, B. Metabolic actions of insulin in men and women. *Nutrition* **2010**, *26*, 686–693. [CrossRef] [PubMed]
14. Lafontan, M.; Langin, D. Lipolysis and lipid mobilization in human adipose tissue. *Prog. Lipid Res.* **2009**, *48*, 275–297. [CrossRef]
15. Lewis, G.F.; Uffelman, K.D.; Szeto, L.W.; Steiner, G. Effects of acute hyperinsulinemia on VLDL triglyceride and VLDL apoB production in normal weight and obese individuals. *Diabetes* **1993**, *42*, 833–842. [CrossRef]
16. Fukagawa, N.K.; Minaker, K.L.; Rowe, J.W.; Goodman, M.N.; Matthews, D.E.; Bier, D.M.; Young, V.R. Insulin mediated reduction of whole body protein breakdown. Dose-response effects on leucine metabolism in postabsorptive men. *J. Clin. Investig.* **1985**, *76*, 2306–2311. [CrossRef]
17. Jiang, Z.Y.; Lin, Y.W.; Clemont, A.; Feener, E.P.; Hein, K.D.; Igarashi, M.; Yamauchi, T.; White, M.F.; King, G.L. Characterization of selective resistance to insulin signaling in the vasculature of obese Zucker (fa/fa) rats. *J. Clin. Investig.* **1999**, *104*, 447–457. [CrossRef]
18. Perseghin, G.; Scifo, P.; Pagliato, E.; Battezzati, A.; Benedini, S.; Soldini, L.; Testolin, G.; Del Maschio, A.; Luzi, L. Gender factors affect fatty acids-induced insulin resistance in non obese humans: Effects of oral steroidal contraception. *J. Clin. Endocrinol. Metab.* **2001**, *86*, 3188–3196.
19. Amiel, S.A.; Maran, A.; Powrie, J.K.; Umpleby, A.M.; Macdonald, I.A. Gender differences in counterregulation to hypoglycaemia. *Diabetologia* **1993**, *36*, 460–464. [CrossRef]
20. Diamond, M.P.; Simonson, D.C.; DeFronzo, R.A. Menstrual cyclicity has a profound effect on glucose homeostasis. *Fertil. Steril.* **1989**, *52*, 204–208. [CrossRef]
21. Wada, T.; Hori, S.; Sugiyama, M.; Fujisawa, E.; Nakano, T.; Tsuneki, H.; Nagira, K.; Saito, S.; Sasaoka, T. Progesterone inhibits glucose uptake by affecting diverse steps of insulin signaling in 3T3-L1 adipocytes. *Am. J. Physiol. Endocrinol. Metab.* **2010**, *298*, E881–E888. [CrossRef] [PubMed]
22. Zang, H.; Carlström, K.; Arner, P.; Hirschberg, A.L. Effects of treatment with testosterone alone or in combination with estrogen on insulin sensitivity in postmenopausal women. *Fertil. Steril.* **2006**, *86*, 136–144. [CrossRef] [PubMed]
23. Shadid, S.; Kanaley, J.A.; Sheehan, M.T.; Jensen, M.D. Basal and insulin-regulated free fatty acid andglucose metabolism in humans. *Am. J. Physiol. Endocrinol. Metab.* **2007**, *292*, E1770–E1774. [CrossRef] [PubMed]

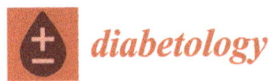

Review

Sexual Dysfunction in Diabetic Women: An Update on Current Knowledge

Federica Barbagallo, Laura M. Mongioì *, Rossella Cannarella, Sandro La Vignera, Rosita A. Condorelli and Aldo E. Calogero

Department of Clinical and Experimental Medicine, Policlinico "G. Rodolico", University of Catania, 95123 Catania, Italy; federica.barbagallo11@gmail.com (F.B.); rossella.cannarella@phd.unict.it (R.C.); sandrolavignera@unict.it (S.L.V.); rosita.condorelli@unict.it (R.A.C.); acaloger@unict.it (A.E.C.)
* Correspondence: lauramongioi@hotmail.it

Received: 13 August 2020; Accepted: 4 September 2020; Published: 10 September 2020

Abstract: Diabetes mellitus (DM) is one of the most common chronic diseases worldwide and its prevalence is expected to increase in the coming years. Therefore, updated knowledge of all diabetic complications and their management is essential for the proper treatment of these patients. Sexual dysfunctions are one of the long-term complications of DM in both genders. However, female sexuality is still a taboo and sexual concerns are often overlooked, underdiagnosed, and untreated. The aim of this review is to summarize the current knowledge on the relationship between sexual function and DM in women. In particular, we evaluated the prevalence, etiology, diagnostic approaches, and current treatment options of female sexual dysfunction (FSD) in diabetic patients.

Keywords: female sexual dysfunction; sexual health; sexual distress; diabetes; hyperglycemia

1. Introduction

Diabetes mellitus (DM) is one of the most common chronic diseases worldwide. The global diabetes prevalence in 2019 has been estimated to be 9.3% (463 million people) and this number is expected to increase by 25% in 2030 and by 51% in 2045 [1]. DM is associated with many long-term systemic complications among which sexual dysfunction is one of them in both genders. In recent years, this aspect has been more extensively studied in men than in women. Sexual dysfunctions in diabetic women are often overlooked due to social taboos on female sexuality [2]. Nevertheless, the analysis of the National Health and Social Life Survey showed that sexual dysfunctions are more frequent in women (43%) than in men (31%) in the US population [3]. In recent years, the attention on female sexual dysfunction (FSD) has been growing. The World Health Organization (WHO) declared female sexuality to be not only part of health quality but also a basic human right [4]. Therefore, the aim of this review is to summarize the current knowledge on the relationship between sexual health and DM in women. In detail, we evaluated the prevalence, etiology, diagnostic approaches, and treatment options of FSD in diabetic women.

2. Physiology of the Female Sexual Response

Masters and Johnson first described the physiological responses to sexual stimulation in their book *Human Sexual Response*, published in 1966 [5]. According to their model, the female sexual response can be divided into four phases: excitement, plateau, orgasm, and resolution. At the same time, later, Kaplan introduced the aspect of "desire" and proposed a three-phase model consisting of desire, arousal, and orgasm [6]. However, women often describe an overlapping of sexual response phases in a variable order. Therefore, more recently, Basson suggested that the female sexual response is not a linear progression of phases but it can be considered a circular sex response cycle with overlapping phases. This model also introduced the importance of multiple psychosocial factors such as emotional intimacy, satisfaction with the relationship, self-image, and earlier negative sexual experience, which can significantly impair female sexuality [7].

Sexual desire is regulated by the effects of various neurotransmitters. Upon activation of the central nervous system and related limbic-hippocampal structures responsible for sexual arousal, electrical signals are transmitted through the parasympathetic and sympathetic nervous system. During sexual arousal, genital vasocongestion occurs as a result of increased blood flow. Increased blood flow to the clitoral cavernosal and labial arteries results in increased clitoral intracavernous tumescence, and engorgement and eversion of the labia minora. The vaginal canal is lubricated and it dilates as a result of relaxation of the vaginal wall smooth muscle [8]. Thus, as in men, sexual response is a neurovascular-dependent event. Previous studies have shown that the nitric oxide-cyclic guanosine monophosphate–phosphodiesterase type 5 pathway plays a pivotal role in modulating blood flow and smooth muscle relaxation in both clitoris and vagina [9]. The vasoactive intestinal polypeptide (VIP) and nitric oxide (NO) are nonadrenergic/noncholinergic neurotransmitters (NANC) which are involved in modulating vaginal relaxation and secretory processes. Moreover, sexual hormones play a significant role in regulating female sexual function [8].

3. Female Sexual Dysfunction

Many studies report a high prevalence of sexual dysfunctions in women. In contrast, FSD is often undiagnosed and almost always undertreated [10]. Thus, data on the real prevalence of FSD are difficult to obtain and they are generally underestimated. According to the data of "The Prevalence of Female Sexual Problems Associated with Distress and Determinants of Treatment Seeking (PRESIDE) study", involving 31,581 US women, sexual problems (desire, arousal, and orgasm) affect 43.1% of women. Hypoactive sexual desire is the most common dysfunction reported by 39% of women, low arousal by 26%, and orgasm problems by 21% [11]. In Europe, the "Women's International Sexuality and Health Survey" (WISHeS), conducted in 1356 women from Germany, United Kingdom, France, and Italy, reported a prevalence of FSD in 29% of women [12].

FSD is a heterogeneous group of disorders that can be related to desire, arousal, orgasm, or sexual pain [13]. During the last decades, several definitions and classifications of FSD have been proposed. Figure 1 reports the history of the main classifications of FSD and the main classifications of FSD are described in Table 1.

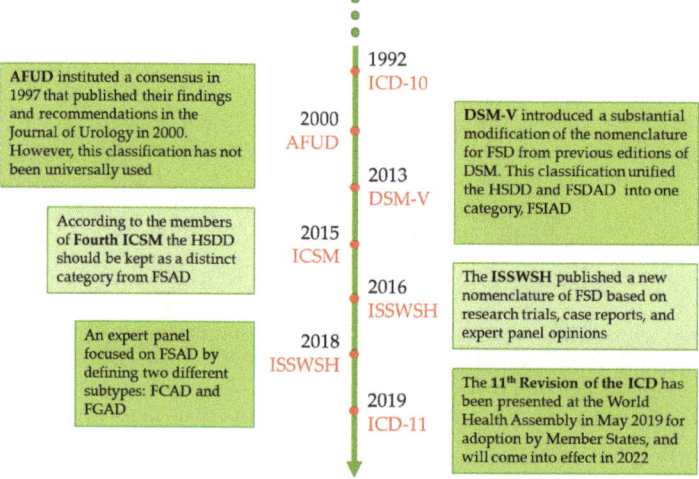

Figure 1. History of the main classifications of female sexual dysfunctions.

Table 1. The main classifications of female sexual dysfunctions proposed during the past decades.

ICD		DSM	ICSM	ISSWSH	
ICD-10	ICD-11 (Proposed)	DSM-V	Fourth ICSM	ISSWSH-2016	ISSWSH-2018
1. Lack or loss of sexual desire	Hypoactive sexual desire dysfunction	1. Female sexual interest/arousal disorder	1. Hypoactive sexual desire dysfunction	1. Hypoactive sexual desire disorder	1. Hypoactive sexual desire disorder
2. Sexual aversion	Recommended for deletion	2. Female orgasmic disorder	2. Female sexual arousal dysfunction	2. Female genital arousal disorder	2. Female sexual arousal disorder: -Female cognitive arousal disorder -Female genital arousal disorder
3. Lack of sexual enjoyment	Female sexual arousal dysfunction		3. Female orgasmic dysfunction	3. Persistent genital arousal disorder	3. Persistent genital arousal disorder
4. Failure of sexual response		3. Genito-pelvic/ penetration disorder	4. Female genital-pelvic pain dysfunction	4. Female orgasm disorders	4. Female orgasm disorders
5. Orgasmic dysfunction	Orgasmic dysfunction		5. Persistent genital arousal disorder	5. Female orgasmic illness syndrome	5. Female orgasmic illness syndrome
6. Non organic vaginismus	Sexual pain penetration disorder		6. Postcoital syndrome (Postorgasmic illness syndrome)		

ICD: International Classification of Diseases and Related Health Problems. DSM: Diagnostic and Statistical Manual of Mental Disorders. ICSM: International Consultation on Sexual Medicine. ISSWSH: International Society for the Study of Women's Sexual Health.

According to the current epidemiology, the more recent classifications International Consultation on Sexual Medicine (ICSM), ISSWH, and ICD-11 suggest that the hypoactive sexual desire should be kept as a distinct category from the dysfunction of female sexual arousal [14]. Moreover, in recent years, sexual distress has become a key element for the definition and the diagnosis of FSD. It can be manifest as thoughts of concern, frustration, hopelessness, or distressing behaviors such as avoidance of sexual situations [14]. The International Classification of Diseases and Related Health Problems, 10th Edition (ICD-10), published in 1992, and the Diagnostic and Statistical Manual of Mental Disorders, Fifth Edition (DSM-5) by the American Psychiatric Association, published in 2013, have been widely used internationally. The 11th Revision of the ICD contains a new chapter on disorders related to sexual health in which modifiable psychological factors do not exclude the diagnosis of sexual dysfunction [15]. ICD-11 has been presented at the World Health Assembly in May 2019 for adoption by Member States, and will come into effect in 2022. In 2015, expert members of the Fourth International Consultation on Sexual Medicine (ICSM) reviewed previous classifications and proposed a new version. In 2016 the International Society for the Study of Women's Sexual Health (ISSWSH) published a new nomenclature of FSD based on research trials, case reports, and expert panel opinions [16]. An expert panel focused on sexual arousal disorders in women (FSAD) convened in February 2018. This panel revised the ISSWSH nomenclature published in 2016 to include female cognitive arousal disorder (FCAD) and modify the definition of female genital arousal disorder (FGAD), two subtypes of FSAD [13].

4. Sexual Dysfunctions in Women with Diabetes Mellitus

4.1. Epidemiology

Data on the prevalence of FSD in diabetic women are few and often discordant because of the lack of standardization in methods and the ongoing changes in FSD definitions and classifications [17]. However, previous studies have shown a higher prevalence of FSD in diabetic compared to nondiabetic women [18]. A meta-analysis showed a higher frequency of FSD in diabetic women than in healthy controls with an odds ratio of 2.27 in type 1 diabetes (DM1), 2.49 in type 2 diabetes (DM2), and 2.02 when considering any form of diabetes [19]. Another Italian study has shown a significantly higher prevalence of FSD in women with DM1 than in the control group (36.4% vs. 5.2%, respectively) [17]. According to a recent meta-analysis, involving 25 studies and 3892 women with an age range of 18–72 years, the overall prevalence of FSD in women DM2 was 68.6% (95% CI 61.6–75.3%) [2]. Results of meta-regression analysis have also shown a statistically significant increase in FSD prevalence in diabetic women over the years [2]. All the phases of sexual cycle response, including desire, arousal, lubrication, orgasm, and satisfaction, are impaired in diabetic women. Meeking and colleagues described a reduction in sexual desire (64%), loss of vaginal lubrication (70%), difficulty of achieving orgasm (50%), decrease satisfaction (47%), loss of genital sensation (36%), and dyspareunia (43%) in 270 women with diabetes aged 21–65 [20].

4.2. Pathogenesis

The pathogenesis of FSD in diabetic women is complex and multifactorial including both psychological and organic causes.

4.2.1. Psychological Factors

In contrast to diabetic men, several epidemiological studies have shown that psychosocial factors are more important than organic factors in the pathogenesis of FSD in both DM1 [21] and DM2 [22]. Diabetic patients have an increased risk to develop depressive symptoms compared to the healthy population [23]. Depression may significantly impair the quality of life of these patients, including sexual function [24]. Therefore, depression is recognized as the most significant risk factor for FSD in diabetic women and it may impair sexual health at different levels.

Sexual dysfunctions can also be side effects of psychopharmacological therapies, such as antidepressants, antipsychotics drugs, mood stabilizers, and anxiolytic drugs [25–27]. Additionally, other psychological problems such as altered self-image, feelings of loneliness, or isolation, loss of attractiveness are common in diabetic women [20]. Several studies have shown a higher risk of FSD in women with higher body mass index (BMI). Although organic factors may have a role in this increased prevalence, an increased BMI can also strongly alter the self-image of women, impairing the quality of sexual life [17].

4.2.2. Organic Factors

Although psychosocial factors seem to have a key role in the pathogenesis of sexual dysfunction in diabetic women, organic factors, including hyperglycemia, neurovascular alterations, hormonal changes, and recurrent genital infections can also contribute to the onset of FSD.

Hyperglycemia decreases the hydration of vaginal mucous membranes, causing a lubrication decrease and, in turn, dyspareunia [20]. Besides, hyperglycemia may increase the risk of vaginal infections [20]. Urinary tract infections (UTI) and mucosal candidiasis are common and often more severe in the diabetic population compared to healthy people [10]. In diabetic women, *Candida albicans* is the most frequent cause of vulvovaginal candidiasis [28]. Hyperglycemia increases the risk not only for incident infection but also for recurrence [28]. Numerous pieces of evidence support the link between lower urinary tract dysfunction and FSD [10]. In particular, the presence of urinary incontinence doubles the risk for decreased libido, vaginal dryness, and dyspareunia [29].

As previously reported, the sexual response is a neurovascular event also in women. It is well known that the chronic insult of hyperglycemia on the endothelium results in endothelial dysfunction. The potential mechanisms involved in endothelial dysfunction include the accumulation of advanced glycation end products, an increase in oxygen-free radicals, and a decreased bioavailability of nitric oxide (NO) [30]. In diabetic men, endothelial dysfunction and the decreased bioavailability of NO result in an insufficient relaxation of the vascular smooth muscle of the corpora cavernosa and in erectile dysfunction [30]. Similar to diabetic men, sexual dysfunctions may be associated with vascular alterations in women with DM. Studies in experimental animals have shown that DM1 alters the contractile and relaxant capacity of vaginal musculature, reduces clitoral and vaginal blood flow, and causes fibrosis of clitoris and vaginal tissue [31–33]. In diabetic women, vascular damage results in decreased vaginal blood, leading to a significantly impaired arousal response [34]. The lack of lubrication is one of the most common sexual problems in diabetic women [19] and it may explain the increased prevalence of dyspareunia, difficulty to achieve orgasm, and hypoactive sexual desire observed in diabetic women compared to healthy controls [19]. A positive relationship between the clitoral pulsatility index with metabolic syndrome and some of its components, especially insulin resistance, has been reported [35]. The pulsatility index is assessed by clitoral eco-color Doppler ultrasound and reflects clitoral vascular resistance to blood flow, which is associated with microvascular lesions [35]. Higher clitoral resistance was also associated with a reduction of sexual arousal, increased anxiety symptoms, and body image concerns [35]. In men, it has been clearly demonstrated that erectile dysfunction is a marker of increased cardiovascular risk [36]. In women, this association is less clear and sexual dysfunctions are not considered an independent marker of increased cardiovascular risk [37]. However, inadequate methodologic tools to explore cardiovascular risks in patients with FSD could have an important role in this gender difference [37].

Moreover, diabetic neuropathy may alter the normal transduction of sexual stimuli, contributing to the pathogenesis of sexual dysfunctions [38]. It has also been hypothesized that unexplained vulvodynia could be a sign of sensory diabetic neuropathy [39].

Steroid hormonal changes can also play a role in the pathogenesis of FSD in diabetic women. Steroid hormones are important to preserve the anatomy and function of female structures involved in sexuality [40]. It has been shown that DM interferes with steroid hormones at different levels. Insulin and insulin-like growth factors can regulate the activities of important enzymes of steroidogenesis, such as aromatase and 3ß-hydroxysteroid dehydrogenase [41,42]. Additionally, insulin and other growth factors stimulate the proliferation of vaginal epithelium in mice and, in the vagina, estrogens up-regulate the expression of insulin-like growth factor 1 [43,44]. Moreover, diabetes is often associated with other endocrine disorders, such as polycystic ovarian syndrome or thyroid diseases, which may contribute to the impairment of sexual function in diabetic women [45].

Regarding the relationship between the type of the therapeutic strategy for DM and sexuality, previous studies have shown a higher prevalence of FSD in women with multiple-dose injection compared to continuous subcutaneous insulin infusion [17,30]. This difference could be related to lower glycemic variability in patients undergoing the latter compared to the former [46]. Recently, Corona and colleagues have investigated the effects of novel antihyperglycemic drugs on the sexuality of both women and men. On one side, the increased risk of genital fungal infections may impair sexual function in both women and men. In contrast, the promising metabolic effects and positive (glucagon-like peptide-1 receptor agonists (GLP1RA) and sodium-glucose type 2 cotransporter inhibitors-SGLT2i) or neutral (dipeptidyl peptidase IV inhibitors-DDP4i) effect on weight could improve the gonadal and sexual function in diabetic patients [10].

4.3. Diagnosis

Recently, the International Society for the Study of Women's Sexual Health has developed a process of care (POC) that provides practical recommendations to diagnose sexual dysfunction in women [14]. This POC is addressed to clinicians with any level of competence in sexual medicine and not only to specialists in sexual medicine. Most women find it difficult to talk about their sexual life and would like clinicians to bring up the topic to give them the opportunity to speak about sexual health. For this reason, as first step, the POC recommends a patient-centered communication in which the clinician asks about sexual satisfaction or problems. If sexual dysfunction is identified, a four-step model is proposed. This includes eliciting the story, naming/reframing attention to the problem, empathic witnessing of the patient's distress and the problem's impact, and referral or assessment and treatment. The aim of this communication is to discover the negative effect that the problem is having on the woman's life. In fact, distress is a key element for the diagnosis of FSD, as emphasized by the more recent classifications [14].

Self-administered questionnaires can be very useful. The Female Sexual Function Index (FSFI-19) is one of the most used psychometric diagnostic tests to identify FSD [47]. A reliable short version of this questionnaire, FSFI-6, is well validated for the screening of sexual dysfunction in women. It includes six domains: desire, arousal, lubrication, orgasm, satisfaction, and dyspareunia. The score for each question ranges from 0 or 1 to 5. A total score of ≤19 allows identifying those women who need further investigation, including the full version FSFI-19 and a patient-centered interviewing [48]. In addition, another version of the FSFI-6, the Female Sexual Dysfunction Index-6 (FSDI-6), has been recently developed [49]. A question on the interest in having a satisfying sex life was added in FSDI-6 to better investigate the level of distress that may arise from the identified sexual problems.

Since women with sexual dysfunctions have a decreased perception of the orgasmic intensity compared to healthy women, recently, a new quick and easy psychometric tool, the Orgasmometer-F, has been validated for measuring the orgasmic intensity in women [50].

A physical examination should be performed to identify potential contributing factors including infections, inflammatory, atrophy, and neoplasms [14].

However, if objective investigation methods such as dynamic penile echo color Doppler can be used in men with erectile dysfunction, objective diagnostic approaches are rarely performed in clinical practice for women [37]. This inadequate evaluation of FSD is one of the main factors responsible for the lack of association between sexual dysfunction and cardiovascular health in women [37]. The main marker of sexual arousal is the increase in blood flow in the genital region. Therefore, during the years, different diagnostic systems have been validated to study the blood flow in female genitalia, including indirect measures of heat dissipation (vaginal thermistors, labial thermistor, heated oxygen electrode), vaginal photoplethysmography (VPP), and Doppler ultrasonography [37]. VPP is one of the most used tools to evaluate genital arousal in women. It consists of a clear acrylic, tampon-shaped device that contains a light source that illuminates the capillary bed of the vaginal wall and the blood circulating within it. A phototransistor detects light and the amount of back-scattered light depends on the transparency of engorged and nonengorged tissue thus, in turn, this is an indirect measure of vasocongestion. The Doppler ultrasonography is a quick and noninvasive technique that provides a real-time assessment of anatomy and blood flow of female genitalia [37]. Women with DM1 showed lower clitoral peak systolic velocity, end-diastolic velocity, and higher resistance index compared with healthy controls. After the administration of 100 mg sildenafil, the mean resistance index significantly decreases, indicating an improvement of the clitoral blood flow [51]. The clitoral pulsatility index (PI) has been correlated with metabolic syndrome and with a subjective decrease of the sexual arousal [49]. During the years, several other methods have been developed to evaluate genital blood-flow-including clitoral VPP, laser-Doppler perfusion imaging (LDPI), dynamic contrast and noncontrast MRI, pudendal arteriogram, or to the assess muscular and neural system-including clitoral electromyography. However, none of these methods is well validated and each method has advantages and disadvantages [52].

4.4. Treatment

No specific guideline is available for the treatment of sexual dysfunction in diabetic women. The change of lifestyle, including weight loss and physical activity, is the first step for the treatment of

FSD in diabetic patients. In fact, overweight/obesity is an established and independent risk factor for sexual dysfunction. Bond and colleagues reported that 60% of obese women seeking bariatric surgery had FSD. They also found that after six months from bariatric surgery the FSFI scores significantly increased (from 24.0 to 29.4) and 68% of women with FSD at baseline resolved their problem [53]. Diabetic women with higher adherence to a Mediterranean diet showed a lower prevalence of FSD compared to women with lower adherence to diet [54]. In an ancillary study of the Look AHEAD, a randomized trial evaluating the long-term effects of an intensive lifestyle intervention (ILI) on cardiovascular morbidity and mortality, overweight/obese women with DM2 were also evaluated for sexual function. Specifically, they evaluated changes in sexual function of 229 women in the ILI group compared with the controls who only received support and education. After one year, women with FSD at baseline had an improvement of their FSFI compared to the control group [55].

Psychotherapy, treatment of depression if present, and an adequate glycemic control also play a pivotal role in the improvement of sexual health [30].

Various pharmacological options may also be used. Hormonal replacement therapy is approved for postmenopausal women [30], whereas the use of androgens to treat FSD is still debated. A meta-analysis including 43 studies and 8480 postmenopausal women showed that testosterone administration is associated with a significant increase in the number of satisfying sexual events (mean difference 0.85, 95% CI 0.52-1.18) and sexual desire (standardized mean difference 0.36, 95% CI 0.22–0.50) [56]. However, oral testosterone was associated with an increase in low-density lipoprotein (LDL), whereas nonoral testosterone did not significantly affect lipid profile [56]. In the same year, a Position Statement on testosterone therapy for women recommend that in postmenopausal women with hypoactive sexual desire disorder (HSDD) with or without estrogen therapy, testosterone exerts a beneficial effect on sexual function at doses within the physiological premenopausal range (Level I, Grade A) [57]. However, although testosterone has been studied for the treatment of FSD for several years, at present, no androgen therapy has been approved for FSD by the Food and Drug Administration (FDA). A recent review of testosterone trials for the treatment of FSD has shown that there are several limitations in these studies, including heterogeneity of the sample enrolled, different instruments to evaluate outcomes, and loss of control for confounders factors. These limitations have a key role in the lack of approval for any testosterone treatment for women in several countries [58]. Phosphodiesterase type 5 inhibitors (PDE5), mediating vascular smooth muscle relaxation and increasing vasodilatation, are a very effective treatment for erectile dysfunction in men. In contrast, few successes have been reported for these drugs in the treatment of FSD [59]. Other pharmacological strategies include ospemifene, a selective estrogen receptor modulator, that has been shown effective for the treatment of vulvovaginal atrophy in postmenopausal women with vaginal dryness [60] or flibanserin, 5-HT1A agonist/5-HT2A antagonist, for women with HSDD [61]. Additionally, several nonpharmacological options can be proposed, including vaginal lasers, lubricants, moisturizers, and pelvic floor physical therapy [14]. The management of sexual dysfunction in diabetic women should be performed by a multidisciplinary team, including a diabetologist, a specialist in sexual health, and psychotherapeutics. Further studies are needed to provide effective therapeutic options for sexual dysfunction in diabetic women.

5. Conclusions

DM is one of the most common chronic diseases worldwide and its prevalence is expected to increase in the coming years. Therefore, updated knowledge of all complications present in diabetes and their management is essential for proper treatment of these patients. Despite sexual dysfunctions being one of the long-term complications in both genders, sexuality in female diabetic patients is still taboo and sexual dysfunctions are underestimated. Data on FSD in diabetic women are few also due to the lack of standardization in methods and the ongoing changes in FSD definitions and classifications. Moreover, in contrast to men, objective diagnostic approaches are rarely performed in the clinical practice for FSD.

Sexuality has a fundamental role in health quality. Thus, information and education of both patients and clinicians on sexual dysfunction are the basis for the appropriate management of FSD. Additionally, clinicians not specialists in sexual health should investigate the sexual dysfunction of their diabetic patients and if a problem is suspected or found, women should be referred to other specialists for further assessment and treatment. In fact, the management of sexual dysfunction in diabetic women should be performed by a multidisciplinary team that includes diabetologists, specialists of sexual health, and a psychotherapeutist.

In conclusion, more attention should be dedicated to this frequent complication of diabetes, adequate methodological tools should be developed for a proper diagnosis and further studies are needed to provide effective therapeutic options for sexual dysfunction in diabetic women.

Author Contributions: Conceptualization, F.B. and L.M.M.; methodology, L.M.M. and A.E.C.; data curation, R.C., R.A.C. and S.L.V.; writing—original draft preparation, F.B.; writing—review and editing, F.B. and L.M.M.; supervision, A.E.C. All authors have read and agreed to the published version of the manuscript.

Funding: This research did not receive any specific grant from any funding agency in the public, commercial or not-for-profit sector.

Conflicts of Interest: The authors declare that there are no conflicts of interest that could be perceived as prejudicing the impartiality of the research reported.

References

1. Saeedi, P.; Petersohn, I.; Salpea, P.; Malanda, B.; Karuranga, S.; Unwin, N.; Colagiuri, S.; Guariguata, L.; Motala, A.A.; Ogurtsova, K.; et al. IDF Diabetes Atlas Committee. Global and regional diabetes prevalence estimates for 2019 and projections for 2030 and 2045: Results from the International Diabetes Federation Diabetes Atlas, 9th edition. *Diabetes Res. Clin. Pract.* **2019**, *157*, 107843. [CrossRef] [PubMed]
2. Rahmanian, E.; Salari, N.; Mohammadi, M.; Jalali, R. Evaluation of sexual dysfunction and female sexual dysfunction indicators in women with type 2 diabetes: A systematic review and meta-analysis. *Diabetol. Metab. Syndr.* **2019**, *11*, 73. [CrossRef] [PubMed]
3. Laumann, E.O.; Paik, A.; Rosen, R.C. Sexual dysfunction in the United States: Prevalence and predictors. *JAMA* **1999**, *281*, 537–544. [CrossRef] [PubMed]
4. Gülmezoglu, A.M.; Souza, J.P.; Khanna, J.; Carroli, G.; Hofmeyr, G.J.; Wolomby-Molombo, J.J.; Mittal, S.; Lumbiganon, P.; Cheng, L. The WHO Reproductive Health Library: A Cochrane window on sexual and reproductive health. *Cochrane Database Syst. Rev.* **2013**, *10*, ED000070. [CrossRef]
5. Masters, E.H.; Johnson, V.E. *Human Sexual Response*; Little Brown & Co.: Boston, MA, USA, 1966.
6. Kaplan, H.S. *The New Sex Therapy*; Bailliere Tindall: London, UK, 1974.
7. Basson, R. Women's sexual dysfunction: Revised and expanded definitions. *CMAJ* **2005**, *172*, 1327–1333. [CrossRef]
8. Berman, J.R. Physiology of female sexual function and dysfunction. *Int. J. Impot. Res.* **2005**, *17* (Suppl. 1), S44–S51. [CrossRef]
9. D'Amati, G.; di Gioia, C.R.; Bologna, M.; Giordano, D.; Giorgi, M.; Dolci, S.; Jannini, E.A. Type 5 phosphodiesterase expression in the human vagina. *Urology* **2002**, *60*, 191–195. [CrossRef]
10. Corona, G.; Isidori, A.M.; Aversa, A.; Bonomi, M.; Ferlin, A.; Foresta, C.; La Vignera, S.; Maggi, M.; Pivonello, R.; Vignozzi, L.; et al. Male and female sexual dysfunction in diabetic subjects: Focus on new antihyperglycemic drugs. *Rev. Endocr. Metab. Disord.* **2020**, *21*, 57–65. [CrossRef]
11. Shifren, J.L.; Monz, B.U.; Russo, P.A.; Segreti, A.; Johannes, C.B. Sexual problems and distress in United States women: Prevalence and correlates. *Obstet Gynecol.* **2008**, *112*, 970–978. [CrossRef]
12. Dennerstein, L.; Koochaki, P.; Barton, I.; Graziottin, A. Hypoactive sexual desire disorder in menopausal women: A survey of Western European women. *J. Sex. Med.* **2006**, *3*, 212–222. [CrossRef]
13. Parish, S.J.; Meston, C.M.; Althof, S.E.; Clayton, A.H.; Goldstein, I.; Goldstein, S.W.; Heiman, J.R.; McCabe, M.P.; Segraves, R.T.; Simon, J.A. Toward a more evidence-based nosology and nomenclature for female sexual dysfunctions-part III. *J. Sex. Med.* **2019**, *16*, 452–462. [CrossRef] [PubMed]

14. Parish, S.J.; Hahn, S.R.; Goldstein, S.W.; Giraldi, A.; Kingsberg, S.A.; Larkin, L.; Minkin, M.J.; Brown, V.; Christiansen, K.; Hartzell-Cushanick, R.; et al. The international society for the study of women's sexual health process of care for the identification of sexual concerns and problems in women. *Mayo Clin. Proc.* **2019**, *94*, 842–856. [CrossRef] [PubMed]
15. Reed, G.M.; Drescher, J.; Krueger, R.B.; Atalla, E.; Cochran, S.D.; First, M.B.; Cohen-Kettenis, P.T.; Arango-de Montis, I.; Parish, S.J.; Cottler, S.; et al. Disorders related to sexuality and gender identity in the ICD-11: Revising the ICD-10 classification based on current scientific evidence, best clinical practices, and human rights considerations. *World Psychiatry* **2016**, *15*, 205–221. [CrossRef]
16. Parish, S.J.; Goldstein, A.T.; Goldstein, S.W.; Goldstein, I.; Pfaus, J.; Clayton, A.H.; Giraldi, A.; Simon, J.A.; Althof, S.E.; Bachmann, G.; et al. Toward a more evidence-based nosology and nomenclature for female sexual dysfunctions: Part II. *J. Sex. Med.* **2016**, *13*, 1888–1906. [CrossRef] [PubMed]
17. Zamponi, V.; Mazzilli, R.; Bitterman, O.; Olana, S.; Iorio, C.; Festa, C.; Giuliani, C.; Mazzilli, F.; Napoli, A. Association between type 1 diabetes and female sexual dysfunction. *BMC Womens Health* **2020**, *20*, 73. [CrossRef] [PubMed]
18. Cortelazzi, D.; Marconi, A.; Guazzi, M.; Cristina, M.; Zecchini, B.; Veronelli, A.; Cattalini, C.; Innocenti, A.; Bosco, G.; Pontiroli, A.E. Sexual dysfunction in pre-menopausal diabetic women: Clinical, metabolic, psychological, cardiovascular, and neurophysiologic correlates. *Acta Diabetol.* **2013**, *50*, 911–917. [CrossRef]
19. Pontiroli, A.E.; Cortelazzi, D.; Morabito, A. Female sexual dysfunction and diabetes: A systematic review and meta-analysis. *J. Sex. Med.* **2013**, *10*, 1044–1051. [CrossRef]
20. Meeking, D.R.; Fosbury, J.A.; Cummings, M.H. Sexual dysfunction and sexual health concerns in women with diabetes. *Pract. Diabetes* **2013**, *30*, 327–331. [CrossRef]
21. Enzlin, P.; Mathieu, C.; Van Den Bruel, A.; Vanderschueren, D.; Demyttenaere, K. Prevalence and predictors of sexual dysfunction in patients with type 1 diabetes. *Diabetes Care* **2003**, *26*, 409–414. [CrossRef]
22. Esposito, K.; Maiorino, M.I.; Bellastella, G.; Giugliano, F.; Romano, M.; Giugliano, D. Determinants of female sexual dysfunction in type 2 diabetes. *Int. J. Impot. Res.* **2010**, 179–184. [CrossRef]
23. Schram, M.T.; Baan, C.A.; Pouwer, F. Depression and quality of life in patients with diabetes: A systematic review from the European depression in diabetes (EDID) research consortium. *Curr. Diabetes Rev.* **2009**, *5*, 112–119. [CrossRef] [PubMed]
24. Kennedy, S.H.; Rizvi, S. Sexual dysfunction, depression, and the impact of antidepressants. *J. Clin. Psychopharmacol.* **2009**, *29*, 157–164. [CrossRef] [PubMed]
25. La Torre, A.; Giupponi, G.; Duffy, D.; Conca, A. Sexual dysfunction related to psychotropic drugs: A critical review—Part I: Antidepressants. *Pharmacopsychiatry* **2013**, *46*, 191–199. [CrossRef] [PubMed]
26. La Torre, A.; Conca, A.; Duffy, D.; Giupponi, G.; Pompili, M.; Grözinger, M. Sexual dysfunction related to psychotropic drugs: A critical review part II: Antipsychotics. *Pharmacopsychiatry* **2013**, *46*, 201–208. [CrossRef] [PubMed]
27. La Torre, A.; Giupponi, G.; Duffy, D.M.; Pompili, M.; Grözinger, M.; Kapfhammer, H.P.; Conca, A. Sexual dysfunction related to psychotropic drugs: A critical review. Part III: Mood stabilizers and anxiolytic drugs. *Pharmacopsychiatry* **2014**, *47*, 1–6. [CrossRef] [PubMed]
28. Nyirjesy, P.; Sobel, J.D. Genital mycotic infections in patients with diabetes. *Postgrad. Med.* **2013**, *125*, 33–46. [CrossRef]
29. Rantell, A.; Apostolidis, A.; Anding, R.; Kirschner-Hermanns, R.; Cardozo, L. How does lower urinary tract dysfunction affect sexual function in men and women? ICI-RS 2015-Part 1. *Neurourol. Urodyn.* **2017**, *36*, 949–952. [CrossRef]
30. Maiorino, M.I.; Bellastella, G.; Esposito, K. Diabetes and sexual dysfunction: Current perspectives. *Diabetes Metab. Syndr. Obes.* **2014**, *7*, 95–105. [CrossRef]
31. Park, K.; Ryu, S.B.; Park, Y.I.; Ahn, K.; Lee, S.N.; Nam, J.H. Diabetes mellitus induces vaginal tissue fibrosis by TGF-beta 1 expression in the rat model. *J. Sex Marital Ther.* **2001**, *27*, 577–587. [CrossRef]
32. Park, K.; Ahn, K.; Chang, J.S.; Lee, S.E.; Ryu, S.B.; Park, Y.I. Diabetes induced alteration of clitoral hemodynamics and structure in the rabbit. *J. Urol.* **2002**, *168*, 1269–1272. [CrossRef]
33. Kim, N.N.; Stankovic, M.; Cushman, T.T.; Goldstein, I.; Munarriz, R.; Traish, A.M. Streptozotocin-induced diabetes in the rat is associated with changes in vaginal hemodynamics, morphology and biochemical markers. *BMC Physiol.* **2006**, *6*, 4. [CrossRef] [PubMed]

34. Wincze, J.P.; Albert, A.; Bansal, S. Sexual arousal in diabetic females: Physiological and self-report measures. *Arch. Sex. Behav.* **1993**, *22*, 587–601. [CrossRef] [PubMed]
35. Maseroli, E.; Fanni, E.; Cipriani, S.; Scavello, I.; Pampaloni, F.; Battaglia, C.; Fambrini, M.; Mannucci, E.; Jannini, E.A.; Maggi, M.; et al. Cardiometabolic risk and female sexuality: Focus on clitoral vascular resistance. *J. Sex. Med.* **2016**, *13*, 1651–1661. [CrossRef]
36. Vicari, E.; Di Pino, L.; La Vignera, S.; Fratantonio, E.; Signorelli, S.; Battiato, C.; Calogero, A.E. Peak systolic velocity in patients with arterial erectile dysfunction and peripheral arterial disease. *Int. J. Impot. Res.* **2006**, *18*, 175–179. [CrossRef] [PubMed]
37. Maseroli, E.; Scavello, I.; Vignozzi, L. Cardiometabolic risk and female sexuality-part ii. understanding (and overcoming) gender differences: The key role of an adequate methodological approach. *Sex. Med. Rev.* **2018**, *6*, 525–534. [CrossRef]
38. Duby, J.J.; Campbell, R.K.; Setter, S.M.; White, J.R.; Rasmussen, K.A. Diabetic neuropathy: An intensive review. *Am. J. Health Syst. Pharm.* **2004**, *61*, 160–173; quiz 175–176. [CrossRef]
39. Kalra, B.; Kalra, S.; Bajaj, S. Vulvodynia: An unrecognized diabetic neuropathic syndrome. *Indian J. Endocrinol. Metab.* **2013**, *17*, 787–789. [CrossRef]
40. Semmens, J.P.; Wagner, G. Estrogen deprivation and vaginal function in postmenopausal women. *JAMA* **1982**, *248*, 445–448. [CrossRef]
41. Garzo, V.G.; Dorrington, J.H. Aromatase activity in human granulosa cells during follicular development and the modulation by follicle-stimulating hormone and insulin. *Am. J. Obstet. Gynecol.* **1984**, *148*, 657–662. [CrossRef]
42. Nestler, J.E.; Strauss, J.F. Insulin as an effector of human ovarian and adrenal steroid metabolism. *Endocrinol. Metab. Clin. N. Am.* **1991**, *20*, 807–823. [CrossRef]
43. Ozawa, S.; Iguchi, T.; Takemura, K.K.; Bern, H.A. Effect of certain growth factors on proliferation in serum-free collagen gel culture of vaginal epithelial cells from prepuberal mice exposed neonatally to diethylstilbestrol. *Proc. Soc. Exp. Biol. Med.* **1991**, *198*, 760–763. [CrossRef] [PubMed]
44. Suzuki, A.; Urushitani, H.; Watanabe, H.; Sato, T.; Iguchi, T.; Kobayashi, T.; Ohta, Y. Comparison of estrogen responsive genes in the mouse uterus, vagina and mammary gland. *J. Vet. Med. Sci.* **2007**, *69*, 725–731. [CrossRef] [PubMed]
45. Bhasin, S.; Enzlin, P.; Coviello, A.; Basson, R. Sexual dysfunction in men and women with endocrine disorders. *Lancet* **2007**, *369*, 597–611. [CrossRef]
46. Reddy, M.; Godsland, I.F.; Barnard, K.D.; Herrero, P.; Georgiou, P.; Thomson, H.; Johnston, D.G.; Oliver, N.S. Glycemic variability and its impact on quality of life in adults with type 1 diabetes. *J. Diabetes Sci. Technol.* **2015**, *10*, 60–66. [CrossRef] [PubMed]
47. Rosen, R.; Brown, C.; Heiman, J.; Leiblum, S.; Meston, C.; Shabsigh, R.; Ferguson, D.; D'Agostino, R. The Female Sexual Function Index (FSFI): A multidimensional self-report instrument for the assessment of female sexual function. *J. Sex Marital Ther.* **2000**, *26*, 191–208. [CrossRef] [PubMed]
48. Isidori, A.M.; Pozza, C.; Esposito, K.; Giugliano, D.; Morano, S.; Vignozzi, L.; Corona, G.; Lenzi, A.; Jannini, E.A. Development and validation of a 6-item version of the female sexual function index (FSFI) as a diagnostic tool for female sexual dysfunction. *J. Sex. Med.* **2010**, *7*, 1139–1146. [CrossRef]
49. Maseroli, E.; Fanni, E.; Fambrini, M.; Ragghianti, B.; Limoncin, E.; Mannucci, E.; Maggi, M.; Vignozzi, L. Bringing the body of the iceberg to the surface: The female sexual dysfunction index-6 (fsdi-6) in the screening of female sexual dysfunction. *J. Endocrinol. Investig.* **2016**, *39*, 401–409. [CrossRef]
50. Mollaioli, D.; Di Sante, S.; Limoncin, E.; Ciocca, G.; Luca, G.; Maseroli, E.; Fanni, E.; Vignozzi, L.; Maggi, M.; Lenzi, A.; et al. Validation of a visual analogue scale to measure the subjective perception of orgasmic intensity in females: The orgasmometer-F. *PLoS ONE* **2018**, *13*, e0202076. [CrossRef]
51. Caruso, S.; Rugolo, S.; Mirabella, D.; Intelisano, G.; Di Mari, L.; Cianci. Changes in clitoral blood flow in premenopausal women affected by type 1 diabetes after single 100-mg administration of sildenafil. *Urology* **2006**, *68*, 161–165. [CrossRef]
52. Woodard, T.L.; Diamond, M.P. Physiologic measures of sexual function in women: A review. *Fertil. Steril.* **2009**, *92*, 19–34. [CrossRef]
53. Bond, D.S.; Wing, R.R.; Vithiananthan, S.; Sax, H.C.; Roye, G.D.; Ryder, B.A.; Pohl, D.; Giovanni, J. Significant resolution of female sexual dysfunction after bariatric surgery comparative study. *Surg. Obes. Relat. Dis.* **2011**, *7*, 1–7. [CrossRef] [PubMed]

54. Giugliano, F.; Maiorino, M.I.; Di Palo, C.; Autorino, R.; De Sio, M.; Giugliano, D.; Esposito, K. Adherence to mediterranean diet and sexual function in women with type 2 diabetes. *J. Sex. Med.* **2010**, *7*, 1883–1890. [CrossRef] [PubMed]
55. Wing, R.R.; Bond, D.S.; Gendrano, I.N.; Wadden, T.; Bahnson, J.; Lewis, C.E.; Brancati, F.; Schneider, S.; Kitabchi, A.E.; Van Dorsten, B.; et al. Effect of intensive lifestyle intervention on sexual dysfunction in women with type 2 diabetes: Results from an ancillary look AHEAD study randomized controlled trial diabetes care. *Diabetes Care* **2013**, *36*, 2937–2944. [CrossRef] [PubMed]
56. Islam, R.M.; Bell, R.J.; Green, S.; Page, M.J.; Davis, S.R. Safety and efficacy of testosterone for women: A systematic review and meta-analysis of randomised controlled trial data. *Lancet Diabetes Endocrinol.* **2019**, *7*, 754–766. [CrossRef]
57. Davis, S.R.; Baber, R.; Panay, N.; Bitzer, J.; Cerdas Perez, S.; Islam, R.M.; Kaunitz, A.M.; Kingsberg, S.A.; Lambrinoudaki, I.; Liu, J.; et al. Global consensus position statement on the use of testosterone therapy for women. *Climacteric.* **2019**, *22*, 429–434. [CrossRef]
58. Rowen, T.S.; Davis, S.R.; Parish, S.; Simon, J.; Vignozzi, L. Methodological Challenges in Studying Testosterone Therapies for Hypoactive Sexual Desire Disorder in Women. *J. Sex. Med.* **2020**, *17*, 585–594. [CrossRef]
59. Chivers, M.L.; Rosen, R.C. Phosphodiesterase type 5 inhibitors and female sexual response: Faulty protocols or paradigms? *J. Sex. Med.* **2010**, *7*, 858–872. [CrossRef]
60. Portman, D.; Palacios, S.; Nappi, R.E.; Mueck, A.O. Ospemifene, a non-oestrogen selective oestrogen receptor modulator for the treatment of vaginal dryness associated with postmenopausal vulvar and vaginal atrophy: A randomised, placebo-controlled, phase III trial. *Maturitas* **2014**, *78*, 91–98. [CrossRef]
61. Katz, M.; DeRogatis, L.R.; Ackerman, R.; Hedges, P.; Lesko, L.; Garcia, M., Jr.; Sand, M. BEGONIA trial investigators. Efficacy of flibanserin in women with hypoactive sexual desire disorder: Results from the BEGONIA trial. *J. Sex. Med.* **2013**, *10*, 1807–1815. [CrossRef]

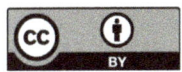

© 2020 by the authors. Licensee MDPI, Basel, Switzerland. This article is an open access article distributed under the terms and conditions of the Creative Commons Attribution (CC BY) license (http://creativecommons.org/licenses/by/4.0/).

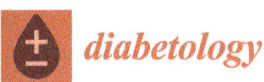

Commentary

Gender Differences in Migration †

Francesca Ena

Ambulatorio Medicina delle Migrazioni, ASL Gallura, 07026 Olbia, Italy; francesca.ena@aslgallura.it
† Proceedings from "Gender differences in diabetes" held in Olbia, 4–5 December 2020.

Abstract: There are about 200 million people on the move in the world, and approximately 50% of them are women. There are no clear migration plans for women leaving as a result of persecution, war, famine, climatic disasters or moving away from contexts of external abuse and even intrafamily violence. Gender-related violence, to which women are exposed in cultural contexts characterized by a patriarchal social organization, is manifested through different ways including, but not limited to, early marriages and genital mutilation, with reproductive health already being seriously impaired at an early age. To this must be added the consideration that low-income countries are not able to deal with chronic degenerative diseases with a multidisciplinary approach such as diabetes. Fragile or non-existent health systems are not prepared for this need, which now affects a third of all deaths from this cause. Compared to Italian mothers, women from high-migration pressure countries had a higher risk of gestational diabetes; in addition, young women of Ethiopian ethnicity are more exposed to increased diabetes risk, in an age- and BMI-dependent way. Gender inequalities are also more evident in migrants for other non-communicable diseases besides diabetes. A major effort is needed in terms of training practitioners and reorganization of basic health services, making them competent in an intercultural sense. Health education of the population as a whole and of women specifically is also needed to contain risk behavior and prevent the early onset of metabolic syndromes in general and of type 2 diabetes in particular.

Keywords: migration; low income; diabetes; gender

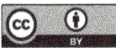

1. Introduction

According to the United Nations International Highlights Report of 2017 [1], there are about 200 million people on the move in the world. Of these, approximately 50% are women. Europe, in particular, is a destination for women who migrate alone, so-called breadwinners, or with a family member, following a plan totally or only partially shared. This migration plan is particularly weak or nonexistent at all for women who leave as a result of persecution, war, famine, climatic disasters or move away from contexts of external abuse and even intrafamily violence. Gender-based violence is heavily present not only in families, but also in social, employment and institutional contexts. We might consider this as a sort of feminization of poverty, becoming one of the strongest push factors that force many young women to leave their country, seeking salvation in completely different contexts. According to the sociologist Mara Tognetti in her review, *"migration is a way to escape cultural references and lifestyles no longer shared"* [2].

As topics related to gender differences in migration are numerous and complex to develop, following the presentation carried out at the meeting "Gender differences in diabetes" (Olbia, 4–5 December 2020), I will mainly address two aspects: (1) motherhood and (2) the greater possibility of the migrant developing diabetes mellitus once they arrive in the host country.

2. Motherhood as a Specific Gender Difference in Migration

Gender-related violence, to which women are exposed in these cultural contexts characterized by a patriarchal social organization, is manifested through labor exploitation, leaving education early, early marriages and even genital mutilation. As a result of this last factor, reproductive health is often already seriously impaired at a very young age. The phenomenon of early marriages is widespread in many countries but reaches significant levels in Central and West Africa, from Chad, where it reaches peaks of 30% in girls under the age of 15, and in Niger, where 70% of girls under the age of 18 go to early marriages, according to the UNICEF report "Achieving a future without child marriage" [3]. Early marriages correlate with school dropout and poor empowerment of young women. Early pregnancies are a direct consequence of this, helping to increase maternal mortality rates and negative outcomes for infants. The practice of female genital mutilation (FGM), spread throughout the equatorial belt and the Horn of Africa, is an emblem of gender violence. It damages the reproductive health of women to different extents, depending on the type to which they are subjected, and interferes heavily with the possibility of living sexually free from physical and psychological conditioning [4,5]. Among the medium- and long-term complications of FGM, obstetric fistula is of note [6,7]. Ischemia from the compression that the head of the fetus exerts during passage in the birth canal, in conditions of protracted dystonia and in the absence of timely obstetric assistance, generates the fistulous tract. The coexistence of some forms of FGM further aggravates the picture, often leading to the death of the fetus. This abnormal pathway allows the passage of feces and/or urine via the vaginal route, resulting in recurrent urinary infections that sometimes result in fatal renal insufficiency. The fate of these women is almost always marked by being victims of social and physical isolation on the part of the family and the community. According to the most recent WHO data, about two million women in sub-Saharan Africa live with this condition and, to this number, about 50–100 thousand cases every year must be added. Gender-based violence continues to undermine the physical and mental health of women, even during migratory routes, at the hands of family members, carers, traffickers, police forces and, unfortunately, even in landing countries. The Global Report on Trafficking in Persons (UNODC 2016) reports that over 75% of people who are victims of trafficking are women, and of these, 20% are minors with a constant global increase in recent years [8]. A large proportion (some 80%) of women victims of trafficking intercepted in Italy come from Nigeria, after having stopped in Libya, a country in which they have suffered further forms of physical and sexual violence, exposed to unwanted pregnancies, induced abortions and sexually transmitted diseases [9,10]. According to the 2018 Action Aid Report—Connected Worlds—the most significant push factor towards Europe, in the case of Nigerian girls, is gender violence.

For some of these women, the degree of awareness with respect to the purpose of migration is clear, but unfortunately, the capacity of aging and empowerment of most of them is almost nil. This inability is also the result of some rituals, such as voodoo practices, to which they are subjected in the country of origin, with the threat of serious consequences on their physical and mental safety as well as that of their family. These observations, although not supported by bibliographical references, originate from the structured interviews conducted with migrant women with an Intercultural Mediator that have made it possible to understand these mechanisms.

Starting street prostitution, with all the risks associated with it, almost always represents the wall against which the migratory plans of the female victims of trafficking are shattered. In this context, another act of violence against these victims is performed: the institutional violence on the part of the host countries, often too concerned about the protection of their borders rather than recognition of the precarious situation in which migrant women are, in particular when they are victims of trafficking. The lack of cultural skills and the condition of isolation that they undergo make it difficult for them to access and correctly use the health services of the host country. This also happens in Italy in the face of a body of legislation that guarantees essential levels of assistance to people in conditions of legal irregularity. The amendment of restrictive provisions such as the Italian Law 132/18 (c.d. Decreto Salvini) has made it more difficult to take charge of and integrate asylum seekers, as pointed out by the Council of Europe: *"the new measures do not offer adequate guarantees to vulnerable persons, such as victims of abuse and torture"*. These restrictive rules, which put the health of already fragile people at risk, only recently have undergone a kind of mitigation, thanks to the advocacy activity of several agencies and scientific societies that, for years, have been dealing with migrant health, in full awareness that poor standards lead to poor health for migrant communities.

The June 2018 editorial of Lancet Public Health "No public health without migrant health" reports what was discussed in Edinburgh, where 700 public health experts from 50 countries produced a statement aimed at soliciting international agencies, governments and public opinion in order to produce different policies about migrant populations and their role in determining their health profile.

Gender, understood not only as genetic sex but as a cultural interpretation of it, is a non-negotiable health determinant in the approach to assessing the health profile of migrant women. From the analysis of Birth Assistance Certificates—Cedap 2016—there are clear differences in access to health services for foreign women, in which the access time to these services is longer than for Italian women, thus reducing the possibility of implementing the now consolidated preventive measures. The Health Observance Report of 2019 confirms that pregnancy and childbirth represent moments of greater contact of foreign women with our health system. In recent years, rates of access have improved in the times recommended by the protocols for taking proper care during pregnancy, as well as the outcomes of newborn children of foreign mothers. However, the persistence of a significant gap between the north and south of the country, with regard to maternal mortality outcomes, cannot be ignored and both neonatal and infantile mortality outcomes follow the historical gap existing in Italy, in terms of health care for the population in general, from the north to the south. The Magazine of the Italian Society of Paediatrics in the article "The unequal Italy begins in cradle" reports alarming data, in particular for the children of women without documents, from sub-Saharan Africa, who have a risk of infant mortality four times higher—8.2/1000—compared to children born from an Italian mother living in the north [11].

Another gender-related issue is the use of voluntary termination of pregnancy, often repeated, by foreign women. Law 194, which regulates access to voluntary termination of pregnancy in Italy, requires that a report be drawn up annually to be submitted to Parliament. From the latest 2020 report, relating to the 2018 data, it is clear that in the face of a trend of continuous decline for Italian and foreign women, voluntary abortion rates persist significantly higher for the latter. It is certain that behind many of these voluntary pregnancy interruptions, there are "hidden" women victims of trafficking. In this complex context, the training of gender-oriented practitioners and the presence of cultural mediators is essential, which, in agreement with each other, can intercept the unclearly expressed needs of foreign women accessing services. The north–south gap in terms of morbidity and fetal maternal mortality correlates with the presence of qualified cultural mediators in the consultations, which are clearly more represented in the north.

In order to improve the quality of access to and proper use of health services by migrant, resident or transiting populations, a number of operational manuals have been published such as guidelines from international and national institutions (OIM-UNHCR, Ministry of Home Affairs, NGO-SIMM-INMP). These guidelines are intended for use by health care professionals, for various reasons, coming into contact with migrant women from the time of landing and on the reception route. Guidelines are very useful for the early detection not only of the disease related to exposure in the countries of origin or acquired in the host country but also for the early detection of women victims of trafficking or FGM. Among the guidelines that are particularly important are those related to the management of victims of intentional physical and/or sexual violence, representing the psychological suffering emerging as pathology among asylum seekers upon reception and, in particular, women exposed to gender violence.

3. Diabetes as a Non-Communicable Disease (NCD) Involved in Migration

In addition to problems related to reproductive health, we cannot ignore that the migrant population are faced with another additional health problem. In fact, especially for those residing in the host country for several years, a so-called epidemiological transition takes place, whereby the health system's focus should be on non-communicable diseases rather than on infectious and imported diseases. Diabetes is a critical issue in the so-called developing countries, where, given the growing population, it is one of the health emergencies from now and in the coming decades, as reported in "Non Communicable Diseases: A Priority for Women's Health and Development" [12]. This increase is particularly significant in the Middle East, North Africa, and sub-Saharan Africa followed by Southeast Asia. The genetic predisposition of some ethnicities and, above all, the forced urbanization with consequent modification of the alimentary habits and acquisition of risk lifestyles (smoke, alcohol, inadequate feeding) are the main reasons for the significant increase in type 2 diabetes in these populations. In this regard, the research carried out on the population of Ovahimba in the North of Namibia is interesting [13]. The authors found that alterations in cortisol homeostasis may link changes in sociocultural environment to increased diabetes and metabolic risk. This work highlights an increase in cortisol secretion related to stress from urbanization, resulting in a diabetogenic effect. In this population, urbanization is associated with an increasing prevalence of disorders of glucose metabolism and other unfavorable metabolic parameters. Besides changes in lifestyle, this may be attributed to an increased cortisol exposure due to living in an urban environment. In another population in Tanzania, an important shift toward an inflammatory phenotype has been associated with an urban lifestyle, providing data on the metabolic factors that may affect diabetes epidemiology in sub-Saharan African countries [14]. It should be taken into account that low-income countries are not able to deal with chronic degenerative diseases with a multidisciplinary approach. Fragile or nonexistent health systems are not prepared for this need, which now affects a third of all deaths from these causes [15,16]. Until now, health care in low-income countries has been based on the support of international donors, sometimes conditional, but focused on vertical interventions for the treatment and prevention of individual infectious diseases (for example, among many, the fight against HIV, tuberculosis, malaria, etc.). Such an approach cannot be transferred to the management of chronic degenerative diseases that cannot be managed with the care of single instants of their natural history. For some years, other intervention models, defined as diagonal, have been tested [17]. These models are capable of implementing strategies identifying priority areas of intervention, which may lead to general improvements in health systems such as the training of local human and professional resources, planning of the use of financial resources and infrastructure, the provision of medicines, and quality of services. This means that interventions intended for a single disease can also have positive effects on preventing and treating other forms of pathology as well as improving the quality of local health systems by overcoming sectoral interventions.

As far as Italy is concerned, the demographic trend towards an ageing population does not spare the migrant population [18]. The migratory phenomenon in Italy is now consolidated if we consider that this migratory balance was reversed in 1973. Currently, in Italy, people arrive at a young age and through their genetic profile, their exposure to strenuous work and unhealthy lifestyles (alcohol, smoking, inadequate nutrition, sedentary lifestyle) makes them prone to chronic degenerative diseases, among which type 2 diabetes plays a prevalent role, sometimes appearing even earlier than in the native population. In our country, the acquisition of Western lifestyles and scarce economic availability mean that, in many families, food of little nutritional value but rich in fat is consumed. The tendency to overweight and obesity in children and unhealthy behaviors such as poor physical activity are now frequent in these subjects. The consumption of sugary drinks does not spare children from migrant families, as shown by the Okkio national health surveillance system of 2016, coordinated by the Higher Institute of Health, where it was reported that in contrast to the observed decrease in childhood overweight and obesity observed in Italian children from 2008 to 2016, this did not apply to migrant children [19]. Compared to Italian mothers, women from high migration pressure countries had a higher risk of gestational diabetes and of all considered adverse events [20]. This is also true for Ethiopian ethnicity, which in Israel, was found to be associated with increased risk of diabetes, in an age- and BMI-dependent way, since young Ethiopians (<50 yrs), particularly women, had the greatest increase in risk [21]. Recently, French authors feared that migrants shared an increased risk of uncontrolled diabetes and, therefore, migration could be a risk factor of uncontrolled diabetes. Knowing the migration history of migrant patients is fundamental to understand certain barriers of care [22]. It has been found that among both Greek-born and immigrant groups, women report substantially higher rates of NCDs, although gender inequalities are more pronounced among immigrants [23].

Human suffering, as a result of natural disasters or conflict, encompasses death and disability from NCD, including diabetes, which have largely been neglected in humanitarian crises [24]. Examining the evidence on the burden of diabetes, use of health services, and access to care for people with diabetes among populations affected by humanitarian crises in low-income and middle-income countries, as well as identifying research gaps for future studies are demanding tasks. The burden of diabetes in humanitarian settings is not being captured, clinical guidance is insufficient, and diabetes is not being adequately addressed. Crisis-affected populations with diabetes face enormous constraints accessing care, mainly because of high medical costs. Further research is needed to characterize the epidemiology of diabetes in humanitarian settings and to develop simplified, cost-effective models of care to improve the delivery of diabetes care during humanitarian crises [24,25].

Since foot lesions can originate from a solitary traumatic event and rapidly progress to gangrene and sepsis, loss of life from diabetic foot infections is both certain and uncounted. Moreover, the problem of diabetic foot disease might be magnified in Africa. The International Diabetes Federation estimates that 70% of Africans with diabetes are undiagnosed. Without a diagnosis, practices known to prevent or mitigate diabetic foot complications will not be implemented and people will die before presentation; this aspect might be amplified by migration, particularly irregular migration [26].

4. Conclusions

A major effort is needed in terms of training practitioners and reorganization of basic health services, making them competent in an intercultural sense. Health education of the migrant population as a whole and of women in particular is needed to contain risk behavior and prevent the early onset of metabolic syndromes in general and of Type 2 diabetes in particular [27]. This also applies to the protection of motherhood in migrant populations.

Funding: This research received no external funding.

Conflicts of Interest: The author declares no conflict of interest.

References

1. International Migration Report 2017 Highlights. Available online: https://www.un.org/development/desa/pd/content/international-migration-report-2017-highlights (accessed on 8 February 2022).
2. Tognetti, M. Donne e processi migratori tra continuità e cambiamento. *ParadoXa* **2016**, *10*, 105–124.
3. Achieving a Future without Child Marriage. Available online: https://www.unicef.org/wca/reports/achieving-future-without-child-marriage (accessed on 8 February 2022).
4. The Global Girlhood Report 2020. Available online: https://www.savethechildren.org/content/dam/usa/reports/ed-cp/global-girlhood-report-2020.pdf (accessed on 12 December 2021).
5. Sciurba, A. Free to choose? The abortion of migrant women in Italy, between migration policies, labor exploitation and extreme cases of abuse and violence. *Int. J. Gend. Stud.* **2014**, *3*, 245–274.
6. Ooms, G.; Van Damme, W.; Baker, B.; Zeitz, P.; Schrecker, T. Diagonal approach to global fund financing: A cure for the broader malaise of health systems? *Glob. Health* **2008**, *4*, 6. [CrossRef]
7. Barry, M.I.; Diallo, I.S.; Bah, M.B.; Cisse, D.; Diallo, T.M.O.; Bah, M.D.; Gnammi, L.R.; Diallo, T.O.; Diallo, K.; Kante, D.; et al. Transection Type, Vesico-Vaginal Fistula Surgery. *Open J. Urol.* **2020**, *10*, 263–274. [CrossRef]

8. Le Donne nei Fenomeni di Migrazione Irregolare, Tratta e Traffico di Esseri Umani. Available online: https://www.academia.edu/37868149/Le_donne_nei_fenomeni_di_migrazione_irregolare_tratta_e_traffico_di_esseri_umani (accessed on 12 December 2021).
9. Krishnan, S.; Dunbar, M.S.; Minnis, A.M.; Medlin, C.A.; Gerdts, C.E.; Padian, N.S. Poverty, Gender Inequities, and Women's Risk of Human Immunodeficiency Virus/AIDS. *Ann. N. Y. Acad. Sci.* **2008**, *1136*, 101–110. [CrossRef]
10. Jaffar, S.; Gill, G. The crisis of diabetes in sub-Saharan Africa. *Lancet Diabetes Endocrinol.* **2017**, *5*, 574–575. [CrossRef]
11. De Curtis, M.; Simeoni, S. L'Italia diseguale inizia in culla. *Pediatria* **2018**, *11*, 18–19.
12. Noncommunicable-Diseases-A-Priority-for-Women's-Health-and-Development Accessed March 2021. Available online: https://ncdalliance.org/resources/noncommunicable-diseases-a-priority-for-women%E2%80%99s-health-and-developmentaccessedmarch2021 (accessed on 12 December 2021).
13. Kann, P.H.; Münzel, M.; Hadji, P.; Daniel, H.; Flache, S.; Peter Nyarango, P.; Wilhelm, A. Alterations of Cortisol Homeostasis May Link Changes of the Sociocultural Environment to an Increased Diabetes and Metabolic Risk in Developing Countries: A Prospective Diagnostic Study Performed in Cooperation with the Ovahimba People of the Kunene Region/Northwestern Namibia. *J. Clin. Endocrinol. Metab.* **2015**, *100*, E482–E486. [CrossRef]
14. Temba, G.S.; Kullaya, V.; Pecht, T.; Mmbaga, B.T.; Aschenbrenner, A.C.; Ulas, T.; Kibiki, G.; Lyamuya, F.; Boahen, C.K.; Kumar, V.; et al. Urban living in healthy Tanzanians is associated with an inflammatory status driven by dietary and metabolic changes. *Nat. Immunol.* **2021**, *22*, 287–300. [CrossRef]
15. Goedecke, J.H.; Mtintsilana, A.; Dlamini, S.N.; Kengne, A.P. Type 2 diabetes mellitus in African women-Web of Science Core Collection. *Clin. Pract.* **2017**, *123*, 87–96.
16. Llácer, A.; Zunzunegui, M.V.; Del Amo, J.; Mazarrasa, L.; Bolu, F. The contribution of a gender perspective to the understanding of migrants' health. *J. Epidemiol. Community Health* **2007**, *61* (Suppl. S2), ii4–ii10. [CrossRef]
17. Lafort, Y.; Lessitala, F.; Ismael de Melo, M.S.; Griffin, S.; Chersich, M.; Delva, W. Impact of a "Diagonal" Intervention on Uptake of Sexual and Reproductive Health Services by Female Sex Workers in Mozambique: A Mixed-Methods Implementation Study. *Front. Public Health* **2018**, *6*, 109. [CrossRef]
18. Baglio, G.; Burgio, A.; Geraci, S. 2019 Health of the Foreign Population–Observation Health. 2020, pp. 334–385. Available online: https://www.ohdsi.org (accessed on 12 December 2021).
19. Lauria, L.; Spinelli, A.; Buoncristiano, M.; Nardone, P. Decline of childhood overweight and obesity in Italy from 2008 to 2016: Results from 5 rounds of the population-based surveillance system. *BMC Public Health* **2019**, *19*, 618. [CrossRef]
20. Seghieri, G.; Di Cianni, G.; Seghieri, M.; Lacaria, E.; Corsi, E.; Lencioni, C.; Gualdani, E.; Voller, F.; Francesconi, P. Risk and adverse outcomes of gestational diabetes in migrants: A population cohort study. *Diabetes Res. Clin. Pract.* **2020**, *163*, 108128. [CrossRef]
21. Jaffe, A.; Giveon, S.; Wulffhart, L.; Oberman, B.; Freedman, L.; Ziv, A.; Kalter-Leibovici, O. Diabetes among Ethiopian Immigrants to Israel: Exploring the Effects of Migration and Ethnicity on Diabetes Risk. *PLoS ONE* **2016**, *11*, e0157354. [CrossRef]
22. Chambre, C.; Gbedo, C.; Kouacou, N.; Fysekidis, N.; Reach, G.; Le Clesiau, H.; Bihan, H. Migrant adults with diabetes in France: Influence of family migration. *J. Clin. Transl. Endocrinol.* **2016**, *7*, 28–32. [CrossRef]
23. Terje AEikemo, T.A.; Gkiouleka, A.; Rapp, C.; Huijts, T.; Stathopoulou, T. Non-communicable diseases in Greece: Inequality, gender and migration. *Eur. J. Public Health* **2018**, *28* (Suppl. S5), 38–47. [CrossRef]
24. Kehlenbrink, S.; Smith, J.; Ansbro, É.; Fuhr, D.C.; Cheung, A.; Ratnayake, R.; Boulle, P.; Jobanputra, K.; Perel, P.; Roberts, B. The burden of diabetes and use of diabetes care in humanitarian crises in low-income and middle-income countries. *Lancet Diabetes Endocrinol.* **2019**, *7*, 638–647. [CrossRef]
25. Boulle, P.; Kehlenbrink, S.; Smith, J.; Beran, D.; Jobanputra, K. Challenges associated with providing diabetes care in humanitarian settings. *Lancet Diabetes Endocrinol.* **2019**, *7*, 648–656. [CrossRef]
26. Rigato, M.; Pizzol, D.; Tiago, A.; Putoto, G.; Avogaro, A.; Fadini, G.P. Characteristics, prevalence, and outcomes of diabetic foot ulcers in Africa. A systemic review and meta-analysis. *Diabetes Res. Clin. Pract.* **2018**, *142*, 63–73. [CrossRef]
27. Kehlenbrink, S.; Jaacks, L.M.; on behalf of the Boston. Declaration signatories: Diabetes in humanitarian crises: The Boston Declaration. *Lancet Diabetes Endocrinol.* **2019**, *7*, 590–592. [CrossRef]

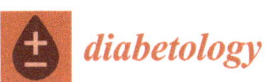

Commentary

Erectile Dysfunction in Diabetic Patients: From Etiology to Management

Rossella Cannarella *, Federica Barbagallo, Rosita A. Condorelli, Carmelo Gusmano, Andrea Crafa, Sandro La Vignera and Aldo E. Calogero

Department of Clinical and Experimental Medicine, University of Catania, 95123 Catania, Italy; federica.barbagallo11@gmail.com (F.B.); rosita.condorelli@unict.it (R.A.C.); carmelo.gusmano@yahoo.it (C.G.); crafa.andrea@outlook.it (A.C.); sandrolavignera@unict.it (S.L.V.); aldo.calogero@unict.it (A.E.C.)
* Correspondence: rossella.cannarella@phd.unict.it

Abstract: Diabetes mellitus (DM) is a widespread chronic disease with a prevalence that is expected to further increase in the near future. The classical management of DM includes the normalization of the glycometabolic profile and the evaluation of cardiac and cerebral vascular health by the intervention of an array of different specialists. However, so far, sexual dysfunctions are still a neglected complication in patients with DM, although there is an elevated prevalence of this long-term complication in male and female patients. Furthermore, some of them may represent a sign of vascular alteration and/or hypogonadism and require timely management to prevent the onset of major adverse cardiac events. This narrative review briefly summarizes the current evidence on epidemiology, pathogenesis, diagnosis, and therapy of erectile dysfunction in male patients with DM to support diabetologists in clinical practice.

Keywords: male sexual dysfunction; sexual health; sexual distress; diabetes; hyperglycemia

1. Introduction

Diabetes mellitus (DM) is a chronic and widespread disease, with a global prevalence of 9.3% in 2019. Worryingly, its prevalence is expected to increase in the near future, by 25% in 2030 and by 51% in 2045 [1]. Several long-term complications are associated with DM, such as diabetic nephropathy, retinopathy, neuropathy, and micro- and macro-angiopathy. Sexual disorders represent one of the neglected long-term complications that can affect both male and female diabetic patients. In men, DM-related sexual dysfunction includes disorders of erection and ejaculation. Their timely diagnosis and proper management would allow not only the increase of the patients' wellbeing and quality of life but can positively impact the primary prevention of major adverse cardiac events (MACEs).

Therefore, this narrative review briefly summarizes the current knowledge of the relationship between sexual health and DM in men. Epidemiological evidence, pathogenesis, diagnosis, and therapy of sexual disorders, mainly focusing on erectile dysfunction (ED) in male diabetic patients, are discussed.

2. Erectile Dysfunction

ED is defined as the persistent failure to achieve or to maintain a penile erection satisfactory for sexual intercourse [1]. Penile erectile structures are the corpora cavernosa, which receive blood supplies by the internal pudendal artery that continues as the penile artery. Corpora cavernosa are made of sinusoids capable of notable volume expansion. Furthermore, they are enclosed in Buck's fascia which rigidly limits their expansion beyond a specific point and this allows the penis to reach its maximal rigidity [2].

A sequential series of events takes place during erection. In the flaccid state, cavernous smooth musculature shows a tonic contraction, allowing only minimal arterial flow for nutritional purposes. When sexual stimulation starts, neurotransmitters are released by the

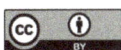

Citation: Cannarella, R.; Barbagallo, F.; Condorelli, R.A.; Gusmano, C.; Crafa, A.; La Vignera, S.; Calogero, A.E. Erectile Dysfunction in Diabetic Patients: From Etiology to Management. *Diabetology* **2021**, *2*, 157–164. https://doi.org/10.3390/diabetology2030014

Academic Editor: Peter Clifton

Received: 29 March 2021
Accepted: 17 August 2021
Published: 4 September 2021

Publisher's Note: MDPI stays neutral with regard to jurisdictional claims in published maps and institutional affiliations.

Copyright: © 2021 by the authors. Licensee MDPI, Basel, Switzerland. This article is an open access article distributed under the terms and conditions of the Creative Commons Attribution (CC BY) license (https://creativecommons.org/licenses/by/4.0/).

cavernous nerve terminals with an ensuing relaxation of cavernous smooth muscles. This leads to the dilation of the arterioles with a subsequent arterial blood flow increase. Sinusoids in turn expand and the subtunical venular plexus is compressed between sinusoids and the tunica albuginea, decreasing the venous outflow [2]. Erection depends upon the parasympathetic nervous system, which causes smooth muscle relaxation by nitric oxide (NO)-mediated action [2].

As known from physiology, the integrity of both vascular and nervous systems is needed for penile erection. Furthermore, NO-mediated erection is dependent on testosterone (T) serum levels [3]. Therefore, the etiology of ED includes psychogenic (e.g., due to stress, depression, or anxiety [4]) and organic forms. The former in turn comprises endocrine causes, such as hypogonadism, hyperprolactinemia, hyper- or hypothyroidism, Cushing's syndrome, Addison's disease, and non-endocrine causes, such as vasculogenic, neurogenic, and/or iatrogenic forms [2].

The vasculogenic etiology includes all the disorders that affect the arterial penile flow (e.g., atherosclerosis, ischemic heart disease, and peripheral vascular disease) and/or the venous outflow (such as venous incontinence, Peyronie's disease, and altered anatomic integrity of the tunica albuginea) [2]. Neurogenic etiology encompasses lesions of the upper motor neuron, sacral lesions, or pudendal nerve injury. Finally, iatrogenic etiology is extended to pelvic surgery and drug intake (e.g., β-blockers, anti-androgens, and luteinizing hormone-releasing agonists and antagonists, etc.) [2].

2.1. Epidemiology

ED has a very high prevalence among the general population. A recent cross-sectional non-interventional study carried out on almost 10 million American men aged >18 years has reported that 573,313 men (~6%) have ED. The prevalence increases from the age of 18 to that of 59, while it decreases in men from 60 to 90 years [5]. Interestingly, patients with ED showed a significantly higher prevalence of cardiovascular disease (CVD) (18% vs. 10%), DM (24% vs. 11%), and depression (11% vs. 5%) compared to patients without ED. The prevalence almost doubled in all these cases [5].

To better explore the association between DM and ED, other studies have assessed the prevalence of ED in patients with DM. A meta-analysis on 145 studies including almost 90,000 patients (mean age 55.8 ± 7.9 years) showed a prevalence of ED of 52.5% in patients with DM, after adjustment for publication bias [6]. Specifically, the prevalence was 37.5% in type I DM (T1DM) and 66.3% in type II DM (T2DM). Furthermore, the studies (n = 17) that used the Sexual Health Inventory for Men (SHIM) questionnaire to diagnose ED showed a prevalence of 82.7%, thus suggesting an even higher prevalence of ED when an accurate diagnostic tool (more than a simple interview) is used [6]. Other evidence collected in patients with DM, reported an age-dependent prevalence of ED, which also correlates with the severity of DM [7].

This evidence strongly highlights the importance of including ED among the long-term complications of DM, and the crucial role of the diabetologist in the early diagnosis of ED in patients with DM.

2.2. Pathogenesis

As previously discussed, several factors are involved in the pathogenesis of ED. Among these, hypogonadism and vasculogenic etiology are of particular relevance in patients with DM. These aspects should be investigated in diabetic patients complaining of ED.

Hypogonadism is often present in patients with DM. A meta-analysis including 37 cross-sectional, longitudinal, or intervention studies, enrolling 1822 T2DM patients and 10,009 controls, reported significantly lower total T (TT) serum levels in patients compared to controls. The same results were found for free-T and sex-hormone-binding globulin (SHBG) levels. Hence, the risk for hypogonadism is greater in patients with DM than in non-diabetic patients [8]. The reason for this association relies on several pathogenetic mechanisms and, in particular, the insulin- and leptin-dependent altered function of the gonadotropin-releasing hormone (GnRH) neuron. Accordingly, GnRH-neuron-secreting activity is influenced by low or high leptin or insulin levels. Insulin receptors are expressed in GnRH neurons but it is not entirely clear whether insulin influences the function of these neurons [9]. In contrast, leptin, released by the adipose tissue, stimulates kisspeptin secretion by the arcuate nucleus that, in turn, triggers GnRH secretion [10]. Patients without diabetes show an obesity-dependent prevalence of hypogonadism and about 33% of obese men have hypogonadism [11]. Similarly, the prevalence of hypogonadism in patients with DM is influenced by the presence of obesity, reaching about 44% in these latter patients [11]. This is of particular relevance, as highlighted by the high prevalence of hypogonadism in patients with so-called "diabesity". Therefore, DM2 increases the prevalence of hypogonadism and the resulting low serum testosterone levels further worsen the health of diabetic patients. This further damages endothelial function since hypotestosteronemia reduces the expression and activity of NO synthase and increases asymmetric dimethylarginine (ADMA) expression [12]. ADMA levels correlate with some cardiovascular risk factors and inflammatory markers, so higher C-reactive protein (CRP) levels are commonly found in patients with DM2 and hypogonadism [13–15]. Finally, hypotestosteronemia modifies, with an androgen-receptor-mediated mechanism, the effects of insulin on the skeletal muscle by decreasing peroxisome-proliferator-activated receptor-γ. This results in higher insulin resistance and worse glycolipid metabolism [16]. The 2020 Standards of Medical Care in Diabetes, released by the American Diabetes Association [17], suggest measuring serum TT levels in patients with DM and symptoms of hypogonadism (e.g., decreased sexual desire or ED). Therefore, diabetologists have a crucial role in the timely diagnosis of hypogonadism. Proper management of hypogonadism is important to improve glycolipid metabolism and cardiovascular health. Indeed, T deficiency has been associated with MACE and independently predicts in-stent restenosis among patients with acute coronary syndrome [18].

In addition to hypogonadism, chronic hyperglycemia activates alternative biochemical reactions, such as non-enzymatic glycation worsening endothelial function. Advanced end-glycation products (AGEs) show direct toxicity as well as receptor-mediated mechanisms, likely involving MAPK-ERK/JNK pathways, in causing vascular damage induced by glycoxidation [19,20].

Moreover, nervous and vasculogenic factors can play a role in the pathogenesis of ED in patients with DM. Microangiopathy causes distress to the vasa nervorum also involving the pudendal nerve that controls erection. A recent multicenter cross-sectional study has positively associated diabetic neuropathy with severe ED in patients older than 65 [21]. Macroangiopathy is an important long-term consequence of DM as well. Since the erection is based on a competent vascular mechanism, the presence of atherosclerotic plaques can lead to arterial ED. The importance of an early diagnosis of a vasculogenic etiology lies in its value as a marker of coronary artery disease, as the so-called "artery size hypothesis" suggests. According to this hypothesis, since the diameter of the penile arteries is smaller than that of the coronary arteries, arteriosclerosis will first show its effects in the small-diameter arteries leading to ED, and subsequently, symptoms of coronary obstruction will follow [22]. Consequently, an early diagnosis of arterial ED can help diagnose the presence of subclinical coronary artery disease if patients are asked to undergo cardiac evaluation. In fact, a systematic review with a meta-analysis on 154,794 patients recently reported a significant increase in the risk of cardiovascular disease, coronary heart disease (CHD), and stroke in patients with ED compared with those without ED. The risk was 43%, 59%, and 34%, respectively [23]. Similarly, a second systematic review with meta-analysis on longitudinal studies, recruiting 92,757 participants followed prospectively for an average of 6.1 years, concluded that there was a significantly higher risk of cardiovascular events in ED patients than in those without ED [24]. Finally, a meta-analysis of observational studies including 22,586 patients reported an odds ratio (OD) of 1.74 for CHD in patients with DM and ED compared to those with DM but without ED [25]. This suggests that the presence of ED further increases the risk for MACE in patients with DM.

2.3. Diagnosis

The diagnosis of ED starts with the patient's interview. When the anamnesis suggests the presence of ED, the administration of a validated questionnaire can be useful to objectively assess its presence and severity. In this regard, the International Index of Erectile Function (IIEF) represents a useful and validated tool [26]. In patients with DM referred for ED, the diagnostic flow-chart should include the evaluation of both TT serum levels and penile echo-color Doppler ultrasound (PCDU) examination after intracavernous injection (ICI).

According to the Endocrine Society, the diagnosis of hypogonadism can be made in the case of TT serum levels below the cut-off of 264 ng/dL (9.2 nmol/L) in at least two different measurements [27]. However, it must be considered that DM has been listed among the conditions that lower either SHBG or TT below the normal range. In these cases, the clinician has to consider that a value of free T < 64 pg/mL (220 pmol/L) confirms the presence of hypogonadism [27].

PCDU examination after ICI with prostaglandin (Pg) E_1 or derivatives (e.g., alprostadil) is a second-line diagnostic test in patients with ED. Despite the lack of standardization of sampling location [28] and cut-off values, a major effort has been made over the decades to identify PCDU waveforms predicting arterial or venous ED [3]. The PCDU allows the measurement of the peak systolic velocity (PSV) and end-diastolic velocity (EDV) of the cavernous arteries in response to ICI drug administration (most often alprostadil). Both of these parameters describe the characteristics of blood flow in the cavernous arteries during erection and are currently used for the diagnosis of vasculogenic ED. Consequently, a restriction of the lumen of the cavernous artery (e.g., due to an arterial plaque or to a greater media-intima thickness) causes arterial blood flow to slow down and the PSV value decreases accordingly. In this regard, a PSV cut-off value between 25 and 35 cm/s is used as the cut-off. Conversely, in the case of dysfunction of the veno-occlusive mechanism (blood is drained too quickly from the dorsal vein of the penis), the EDV increases (>5 cm/s) [3]. In particular, a retrospective study of up to 300 patients with ED followed for 10 years reported that morphological abnormalities of the cavernous arteries (e.g., stenosis, atherosclerotic plaques, and intima-media thickness) were closely associated with cardiovascular disease. In fact, the risk for MACE was three times higher in patients with morphological abnormalities of the cavernous arteries than in those with normal morphology [29]. Once again, this evidence highlights the crucial importance of correct diagnosis and management of ED, given its consequences on cardiovascular health, especially in patients with DM.

2.4. Therapeutic Options

The therapeutic approach to ED differs according to its etiology. Hypogonadism can be overcome after weight loss in patients with "diabesity" [11]. Indeed, weight loss decreases serum levels of leptin, which increases the secretion of kisspeptin and the function of GnRH neurons, thus restoring hypothalamic-pituitary-gonadal function. Consequently, restoration of T levels to the normal range has been reported in obese and hypogonadal male patients after weight loss by prescribing a very-low-calorie ketogenic diet [30]. In the case of overt hypogonadism, testosterone replacement therapy (TRT) may be necessary [27]. In particular, an 11-year-long longitudinal study showed diabetes remission after long-term treatment with injectable T in patients with hypogonadism and T2DM [31].

There are several formulations available that contain testosterone. They include injectable ones consisting of testosterone undecanoate, propionate, phenyl-propionate, isocaproate, decanoate, or enanthate, or a transdermal gel containing testosterone. The oral formulation is little used in clinical practice due to the difficulty of maintaining stable values of serum testosterone due to the variability of its absorption through the intestinal tract.

The choice of the best formulation for TRT depends on patient compliance, as available testosterone-containing available products offer daily, weekly, or monthly administration. Before starting TRT, the risk of prostate cancer and erythrocytosis should be considered. Furthermore, exogenous testosterone temporarily suppresses the hypothalamus-pituitary-testis axis and thus spermatogenesis and fertility. Therefore, TRT should not be prescribed to patients seeking paternity. Alternative treatment is based on the administration of human chorionic gonadotropin [32].

When the cause of ED is vasculogenic, correction of cardiovascular risk factors (e.g., hypertension, hypercholesterolemia, smoking, and obesity) is mandatory. After this step, prescribing phosphodiesterase type 5 inhibitors (PDE5i) is a useful choice. PDE5i acts by hindering the action of the PDE5 enzyme, which in turn increases the bioavailability of NO and cyclic GMP. Several molecules are currently available in clinical practice. These include sildenafil, tadalafil, vardenafil, and avanafil, which differ for bioavailability, pharmacokinetics, affinity, and selectivity for PDE isoenzymes. Sildenafil is mostly used on demand, due to its short bioavailability, while tadalafil can be used daily and could be preferred in patients with contemporary benign prostatic hyperplasia [33]. It is noteworthy that PDE5 is involved in the intracellular signaling of insulin. An in vitro study showed that insulin can stimulate glucose transport via the NO/cyclic GMP pathway in human vascular smooth cells [34]. Furthermore, sildenafil is capable of lowering insulin resistance in human endothelial cells [35]. These findings have led to studies that have assessed the effects of PDE5i on glycemic control in patients with T2DM. The meta-analysis of these studies concluded that sildenafil has no effect on glycated hemoglobin. However, only four studies were included, for a total of only 100 patients with T2DM and 98 controls that were treated with very different doses of sildenafil at various durations [36]. Hence, more evidence based on a greater number of patients and using proper study designs is necessary to better understand the role of PDE5i in the glycometabolic control in patients with DM. Moreover, the benefits of PDE5is have been reported in diabetic cardiopathy, where these molecules can decrease the pro-inflammatory chemokine interleukin-8 [37]. This further indicates the need for a better investigation of the role of PDE5i in patients with DM and ED. Pharmacotherapy also includes local application of alprostadil that can be administered as a topical cream or medicated pellet, both adsorbed via the urethral meatus [38].

Other treatments include vacuum devices, whose efficacy is high but with a slightly increased risk of minor (pain) and major (skin necrosis) adverse events [38,39]. Low-intensity extracorporeal shock wave therapy has been shown to be effective in treating ED by improving the IIEF score and PSV value on the PCDU evaluation [40]. Finally, surgical treatment with inflatable or semi-rigid prosthesis implantation is available for patients who are not responsive to pharmacotherapy or who want a definitive resolution to the problem [38].

3. Conclusions

DM is a chronic and widespread disease whose prevalence is expected to increase in the coming years [1]. Updated knowledge of the complications of this disease is of great importance. However, if some complications are well coded and followed appropriately, sexual dysfunctions and especially ED are not. Nonetheless, ED is a very common complication in male patients with DM. Furthermore, its prevalence increases with advancing age and in patients with long-lasting diabetes and of greater severity, reflecting worse glycometabolic control and worse cardiovascular health. Therefore, an early and timely diagnosis of ED is important to detect the presence of hypogonadism and/or CHD. Correction of cardiovascular risk factors is mandatory in DM patients with ED. Moreover, PDE5is are a useful therapeutic choice, and further studies are warranted to better understand the role of these drugs, if any, in glucose control and cardiovascular health. Taking all these aspects into account, ED can be considered a long-term complication of DM and, in this view, the diabetologist has a pivotal role in its early detection and in the correct management of this aspect (Figure 1).

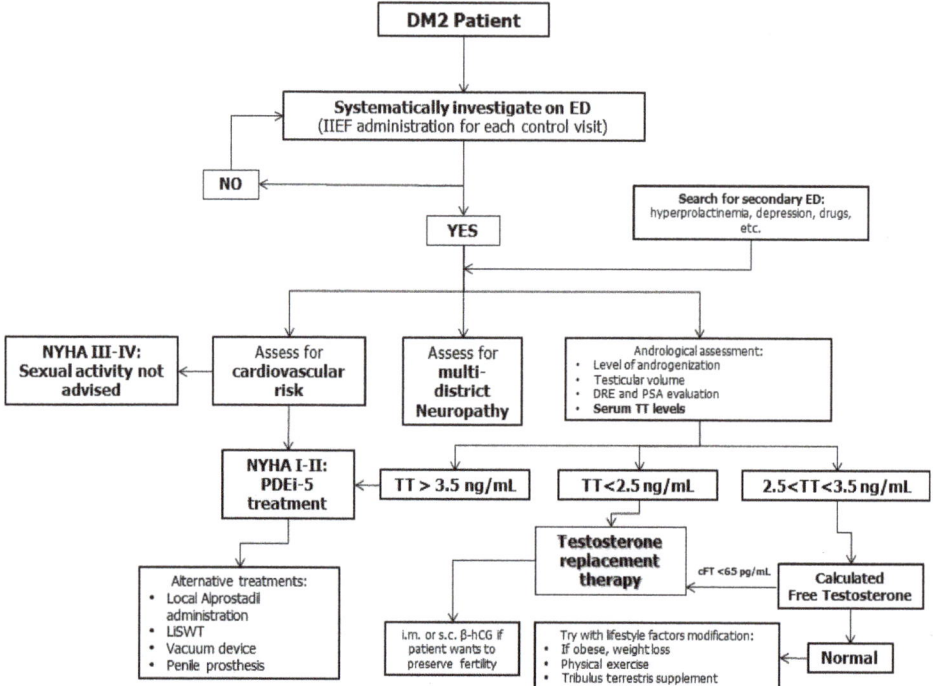

Figure 1. Diagnostic and therapeutic algorithm of erectile dysfunction (ED) management in patients with diabetes mellitus (DM). A systematic evaluation for ED should be carried out in patients with DM. Diagnostic assessment should include evaluation of cardiovascular risk, multidistrict neuropathy, testicular function, and secondary ED. Sexual activity is not recommended in patients with NYHA class III-IV, while treatment can be prescribed in those in NYHA class I-II. Testosterone replacement treatment is indicated in patients with hypogonadism having serum total testosterone (TT) levels consistently below 2.5 ng/mL or between 2.5 and 3.5 ng/mL and low calculated free testosterone.

Author Contributions: Conceptualization, R.C.; methodology, F.B.; data curation, R.A.C. and S.L.V.; writing—original draft preparation, R.C., A.C. and C.G.; writing—review and editing, A.E.C.; supervision, A.E.C. All authors have read and agreed to the published version of the manuscript.

Funding: This research did not receive any specific grant from any funding agency in the public, commercial, or not-for-profit sector.

Conflicts of Interest: The authors declare that there are no conflicts of interest that could be perceived as prejudicing the impartiality of the research reported.

Abbreviations

DRE: digital-rectal exploration; hCG, human chorionic gonadotropin; IIEF-5, International Index of Erectile Function; LiSWT, low intensity shock wave therapy; NYHA, New York Heart Association; PDE5i, phosphodiesterase 5 inhibitors.

References

1. NIH Consensus Conference. Impotence. NIH Consensus Development Panel on Impotence. *JAMA* **1993**, *270*, 83–90. [CrossRef]
2. Calogero, A.E.; Burgio, G.; Condorelli, R.A.; Cannarella, R.; La Vignera, S. Epidemiology and risk factors of lower urinary tract symptoms/benign prostatic hyperplasia and erectile dysfunction. *Aging Male* **2018**, *22*, 12–19. [CrossRef] [PubMed]

3. Zvara, P.; Sioufi, R.; Schipper, H.M.; Begin, L.R.; Brock, G.B. Nitric oxide mediated erectile activity is a testosterone dependent event: A rat erection model. *Int. J. Impot. Res.* **1995**, *70*, 209–219.
4. Cannarella, R.; Calogero, A.E.; Aversa, A.; Condorelli, R.A.; La Vignera, S. Differences in Penile Hemodynamic Profiles in Patients with Erectile Dysfunction and Anxiety. *J. Clin. Med.* **2021**, *10*, 402. [CrossRef] [PubMed]
5. Goldstein, I.; Chambers, R.; Tang, W.; Stecher, V.; Hassan, T. Real-world observational results from a database of 48 million men in the United States: Relationship of cardiovascular disease, diabetes mellitus and depression with age and erectile dysfunction. *Int. J. Clin. Pract.* **2018**, *72*, e13078. [CrossRef]
6. Kouidrat, Y.; Pizzol, D.; Cosco, T.; Thompson, T.; Carnaghi, M.; Bertoldo, A.; Solmi, M.; Stubbs, B.; Veronese, N. High prevalence of erectile dysfunction in diabetes: A systematic review and meta-analysis of 145 studies. *Diabet. Med.* **2017**, *34*, 1185–1192. [CrossRef]
7. Klein, R.; E Klein, B.; E Lee, K.; E Moss, S.; Cruickshanks, K.J. Prevalence of self-reported erectile dysfunction in people with long-term IDDM. *Diabetes Care* **1996**, *19*, 135–141. [CrossRef]
8. Corona, G.; Monami, M.; Rastrelli, G.; Aversa, A.; Sforza, A.; Lenzi, A.; Forti, G.; Mannucci, E.; Maggi, M. Type 2 diabetes mellitus and testosterone: A meta-analysis study. *Int. J. Androl.* **2010**, *34*, 528–540. [CrossRef]
9. Evans, M.C.; Hill, J.W.; Anderson, G.M. Role of insulin in the neuroendocrine control of reproduction. *J. Neuroendocr.* **2021**, *33*, e12930. [CrossRef]
10. Childs, G.V.; Odle, A.K.; MacNicol, M.C.; MacNicol, A.M. The Importance of Leptin to Reproduction. *Endocrinology* **2020**, *162*. [CrossRef]
11. Dhindsa, S.; Ghanim, H.; Batra, M.; Dandona, P. Hypogonadotropic Hypogonadism in Men with Diabesity. *Diabetes Care* **2018**, *41*, 1516–1525. [CrossRef]
12. Tariq, K.; Khan, M.A. Asymmetrical dimethyl arginine in type 2 diabetic patients with coronary artery disease. *J. Pak. Med. Assoc.* **2016**, *66*, 957–960. [PubMed]
13. Wierzbicki, A.S.; Solomon, H.; Lumb, P.J.; Lyttle, K.; Lambert-Hammill, M.; Jackson, G. Asymmetric dimethyl arginine levels correlate with cardiovascular risk factors in patients with erectile dysfunction. *Atherosclerosis* **2006**, *185*, 421–425. [CrossRef]
14. Stühlinger, M.C.; Stanger, O. Asymmetric dimethyl-L-arginine (ADMA): A possible link between homocyst(e)ine and endothelial dysfunction. *Curr. Drug Metab.* **2005**, *6*, 3–14. [CrossRef] [PubMed]
15. Jamwal, S.; Sharma, S. Vascular endothelium dysfunction: A conservative target in metabolic disorders. *Inflamm. Res.* **2018**, *67*, 391–405. [CrossRef]
16. Rao, P.M.; Kelly, D.M.; Jones, T.H. Testosterone and insulin resistance in the metabolic syndrome and T2DM in men. *Nat. Rev. Endocrinol.* **2013**, *9*, 479–493. [CrossRef] [PubMed]
17. Table of Contents. Available online: https://care.diabetesjournals.org/content/43/Supplement_1 (accessed on 30 July 2021).
18. Chmiel, A.; Mizia-Stec, K.; Wierzbicka-Chmiel, J.; Rychlik, S.; Muras, A.; Mizia, M.; Bienkowski, J. Low testosterone and sexual symptoms in men with acute coronary syndrome can be used to predict major adverse cardiovascular events during long-term follow-up. *Andrology* **2015**, *3*, 1113–1118. [CrossRef]
19. Beisswenger, P.J. Glycation and biomarkers of vascular complications of diabetes. *Amino Acids* **2010**, *42*, 1171–1183. [CrossRef]
20. De Nigris, F.; Rienzo, M.; Sessa, M.; Infante, T.; Cesario, E.; Ignarro, L.J.; Al-Omran, M.; Giordano, A.; Palinski, W.; Napoli, C. Glycoxydation promotes vascular damage via MAPK-ERK/JNK pathways. *J. Cell Physiol.* **2012**, *227*, 3639–3647. [CrossRef]
21. Furukawa, S.; Sakai, T.; Niiya, T.; Miyaoka, H.; Miyake, T.; Yamamoto, S.; Maruyama, K.; Ueda, T.; Senba, H.; Todo, Y.; et al. Diabetic peripheral neuropathy and prevalence of erectile dysfunction in Japanese patients aged <65 years with type 2 diabetes mellitus: The Dogo Study. *Int. J. Impot. Res.* **2016**, *29*, 30–34. [CrossRef] [PubMed]
22. Montorsi, P.; Ravagnani, P.M.; Galli, S.; Rotatori, F.; Briganti, A.; Salonia, A.; Rigatti, P.; Montorsi, F. The Artery Size Hypothesis: A Macrovascular Link between Erectile Dysfunction and Coronary Artery Disease. *Am. J. Cardiol.* **2005**, *96*, 19–23. [CrossRef]
23. Zhao, B.; Hong, Z.; Wei, Y.; Yu, D.; Xu, J.; Zhang, W. Erectile Dysfunction Predicts Cardiovascular Events as an Independent Risk Factor: A Systematic Review and Meta-Analysis. *J. Sex. Med.* **2019**, *16*, 1005–1017. [CrossRef] [PubMed]
24. Vlachopoulos, C.; Terentes-Printzios, D.; Ioakeimidis, N.; Aznaouridis, K.; Rokkas, K.; Synodinos, A.; Christoforatou, E.; Aggelis, A.; Samentzas, A.; Stefanadis, C. Prediction of cardiovascular events and all-cause mortality with erectile dysfunction: A systematic review and meta-analysis of cohort studies. *J. Am. Coll. Cardiol.* **2012**, *59*, E2074. [CrossRef]
25. Yamada, T.; Hara, K.; Umematsu, H.; Suzuki, R.; Kadowaki, T. Erectile Dysfunction and Cardiovascular Events in Diabetic Men: A Meta-analysis of Observational Studies. *PLoS ONE* **2012**, *7*, e43673. [CrossRef] [PubMed]
26. Rosen, R.C.; Cappelleri, J.C.; Gendrano, N. The International Index of Erectile Function (IIEF): A state-of-the-science review. *Int. J. Impot. Res.* **2002**, *14*, 226–244. [CrossRef]
27. Bhasin, S.; Brito, J.P.; Cunningham, G.R.; Hayes, F.J.; Hodis, H.N.; Matsumoto, A.M.; Snyder, P.J.; Swerdloff, R.S.; Wu, F.C.; A Yialamas, M. Testosterone Therapy in Men with Hypogonadism: An Endocrine Society* Clinical Practice Guideline. *J. Clin. Endocrinol. Metab.* **2018**, *103*, 1715–1744. [CrossRef] [PubMed]
28. Pagano, M.; Stahl, P.J. Variation in Penile Hemodynamics by Anatomic Location of Cavernosal Artery Imaging in Penile Duplex Doppler Ultrasound. *J. Sex. Med.* **2015**, *12*, 1911–1919. [CrossRef]
29. Caretta, N.; Ponce, M.D.R.; Minicuci, N.; Palego, P.; Valente, U.; Garolla, A.; Ferlin, A.; Foresta, C. Penile doppler ultrasound predicts cardiovascular events in men with erectile dysfunction. *Andrology* **2018**, *7*, 82–87. [CrossRef] [PubMed]

30. La Vignera, S.; Cannarella, R.; Galvano, F.; Grillo, A.; Aversa, A.; Cimino, L.; Magagnini, C.M.; Mongioì, L.M.; Condorelli, R.A.; Calogero, A.E. The ketogenic diet corrects metabolic hypogonadism and preserves pancreatic ß-cell function in overweight/obese men: A single-arm uncontrolled study. *Endocrine* **2020**. [CrossRef]
31. Haider, K.S.; Haider, A.; Saad, F.; Doros, G.; Hanefeld, M.; Dhindsa, S.; Dandona, P.; Traish, A. Remission of type 2 diabetes following long-term treatment with injectable testosterone undecanoate in patients with hypogonadism and type 2 diabetes: 11-year data from a real-world registry study. *Diabetes, Obes. Metab.* **2020**, *22*, 2055–2068. [CrossRef]
32. Corona, G.; Goulis, D.G.; Huhtaniemi, I.; Zitzmann, M.; Toppari, J.; Forti, G.; Vanderschueren, D.; Wu, F.C. European Academy of Andrology (EAA) guidelines on investigation, treatment and monitoring of functional hypogonadism in males: Endorsing organization: European Society of Endocrinology. *Andrology* **2020**, *8*, 970–987. [CrossRef]
33. Sebastianelli, A.; Spatafora, P.; Morselli, S.; Vignozzi, L.; Serni, S.; McVary, K.T.; Kaplan, S.; Gravas, S.; Chapple, C.; Gacci, M. Tadalafil Alone or in Combination with Tamsulosin for the Management for LUTS/BPH and ED. *Curr. Urol. Rep.* **2020**, *21*, 1–12. [CrossRef]
34. Bergandi, L.; Silvagno, F.; Russo, I.; Riganti, C.; Anfossi, G.; Aldieri, E.; Ghigo, D.; Trovati, M.; Bosia, A. Insulin Stimulates Glucose Transport Via Nitric Oxide/Cyclic GMP Pathway in Human Vascular Smooth Muscle Cells. *Arterioscler. Thromb. Vasc. Biol.* **2003**, *23*, 2215–2221. [CrossRef] [PubMed]
35. Mammi, C.; Pastore, D.; Lombardo, M.F.; Ferrelli, F.; Caprio, M.; Consoli, C.; Tesauro, M.; Gatta, L.; Fini, M.; Federici, M.; et al. Sildenafil Reduces Insulin-Resistance in Human Endothelial Cells. *PLoS ONE* **2011**, *6*, e14542. [CrossRef]
36. Poolsup, N.; Suksomboon, N.; Aung, N. Effect of phosphodiesterase-5 inhibitors on glycemic control in person with type 2 diabetes mellitus: A systematic review and meta-analysis. *J. Clin. Transl. Endocrinol.* **2016**, *6*, 50–55. [CrossRef] [PubMed]
37. Giannattasio, S.; Corinaldesi, C.; Colletti, M.; Di Luigi, L.; Antinozzi, C.; Filardi, T.; Scolletta, S.; Basili, S.; Lenzi, A.; Morano, S.; et al. The phosphodiesterase 5 inhibitor sildenafil decreases the proinflammatory chemokine IL-8 in diabetic cardiomyopathy: In vivo and in vitro evidence. *J. Endocrinol. Investig.* **2018**, *42*, 715–725. [CrossRef]
38. Salonia, A.; Bettocchi, C.; Boeri, L.; Capogrosso, P.; Carvalho, J.; Cilesiz, N.C.; Cocci, A.; Corona, G.; Dimitropolous, K.; Gül, M.; et al. EAU Working Group on Male Sexual and Reproductive Health. European Association of Urology Guidelines on Sexual and Re-productive Health-2021 Update: Male Sexual Dysfunction. *Eur. Urol.* **2021**, *25*, S0302-2838(21)01813-3.
39. Beaudreau, S.A.; Van Moorleghem, K.; Dodd, S.M.; Liou-Johnson, V.; Suresh, M.; Gould, C.E. Satisfaction with a Vacuum Constriction Device for Erectile Dysfunction among Middle-Aged and Older Veterans. *Clin. Gerontol.* **2020**, *44*, 307–315. [CrossRef]
40. Sokolakis, I.; Hatzichristodoulou, G. Clinical studies on low intensity extracorporeal shockwave therapy for erectile dysfunction: A systematic review and meta-analysis of randomised controlled trials. *Int. J. Impot. Res.* **2019**, *31*, 177–194. [CrossRef] [PubMed]

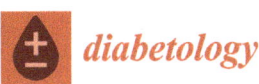

Commentary

Sex-Gender Awareness in Diabetes

Giancarlo Tonolo [1,2]

[1] S.C. Diabetologia, P.O. San Giovanni di Dio, ASSL Olbia-ATS Sardegna, 07026 Olbia, Italy; giancarlo.tonolo@atssardegna.it
[2] JANASDIA Association, 07026 Olbia, Italy

Abstract: Sex and gender can affect incidence, prevalence, symptoms, course and response to drug therapy in many illnesses, being sex (the biological side) and gender (the social-cultural one), variously interconnected. Indeed, women have greater longevity; however, this is accompanied by worse health than men, particularly when obesity is present. Sex-gender differences are fundamental also in both type 1 and type 2 diabetes. Just for example in the prediabetes situation impaired fasting glucose (expression of increased insulin resistance) is more common in men, while impaired glucose tolerance (expression of beta cell deficiency) is more common in female, indicating a possible different genesis of type 2 diabetes in the two sexes. In type 1 diabetes male and female are equivalent as incidence of the disease since puberty, while estrogens act as protective and reduce the incidence of type 1 diabetes in female after puberty. Considering macrovascular complications, diabetic women have a 3.5 fold higher increased cardiovascular risk than non diabetic women, against an observed increase of "only" 2.1 fold in male. Thus it is clear, although not fully explained, that sex-gender differences do exist in diabetes. Another less studied aspect is that also physician gender influences quality of care in patients with type 2 diabetes, female physicians providing an overall better quality of care, especially in risk management. The goal of this short commentary is to open the special issue of Diabetology: "Gender Difference in Diabetes" leaving to the individual articles to deepen differences in genesis, psychologists aspects and complications of the disease.

Keywords: type 1 diabetes; type 2 diabetes; cardiovascular disease; diabetic retinopathy; drug therapy in diabetes

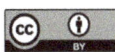

1. Introduction

Diabetes mellitus and cardiovascular diseases act as two sides of the same coin: diabetes is considered as an equivalent of ischemic cardiovascular disease while patients with ischemic cardiovascular disease often have diabetes or pre-diabetes. Diabetic women have a 3.5 fold higher increased cardiovascular risk than non diabetic women, against an observed increase of "only" 2.1 fold in male. Gender is considered as the social expression that transforms a female into a woman and a male into a man, while sex is the set of biological aspects of being female or male. The differences and inequalities in the state of health often derive from both biological (sex) and social-cultural (gender) differences that are variously interconnected, so I prefer to use the term sex-gender in this commentary, as it has been done before [1,2].

In view of the impact of sex hormones on glucose homeostasis and on the molecular pathways involved in insulin resistance, sex-gender specific mechanisms in the development of diabetic complications are more than suspected, but leave an unmet need of specific sex-gender therapeutic approaches.

There is scientific evidence that sex and gender can affect the incidence, prevalence, symptoms, course and response of many illnesses. Women have greater longevity, but this is accompanied by worse health than men, particularly when obesity is present: over the age of 65, women have three or more chronic diseases more often than men and suffer from greater disability [3]. Women have a higher prevalence of psychiatric, musculoskeletal and some autoimmune pathologies compared to men of the same age. Sex-gender differences are fundamental also in both type 1 (insulin dependent, T1DM) and type 2 (non-insulin dependent, T2DM) diabetes.

2. Type 2 Diabetes

Regarding T2DM, sex-gender differences do have a role in the homeostasis of glucose, even in the prediabetic syndromes impaired fasting glucose (IFG), more related to insulin resistance and impaired glucose tolerance (IGT), more related to beta cell dysfunction. IFG is more prevalent in males, while IGT in women is a disease that occurs mainly due to insulin resistance and loss of beta cell function combined together differently [4,5], suggesting clear sex-gender different etiological mechanisms that lead to T2DM. T2DM has a higher prevalence in men, but since women are more numerous, there are more women than men affected [6–8].

Another area of sex-gender difference in glucose homeostasis is the bi-directional modulation of diabetes risk by testosterone in males and females. In males, testosterone protects against diabetes, as hypogonadism induced with anti-testosterone therapy for prostate cancer is reported to promote the development of T2DM. The same applies when physiological age related hypogonadism appears. On the contrary, testosterone administration in hypogonadal males improves insulin sensitivity, and has a multidimensional favorable effect on cardiovascular risk profile. The effects of testosterone are rather different in women. Women with testosterone excess exhibit initial β-cell hyper-function, which may predispose them to secondary β-cell failure and type 2 diabetes [1].

3. Type 1 Diabetes

Regarding T1DM, less is known about sex-gender differences. In any case, T1DM is the only common autoimmune disease with a peak of onset of less than 15 years of age that is characterized by male: female ratio of about 1.5 worldwide, with an incidence of the disease similar between the two sexes until puberty and a decreases in women thereafter, although female T1DM patients have higher levels of GADAab (antibodies against glutamic acid decarboxylase) and a more severe loss of beta-cell function than male patients with the same age at diagnosis. The decrease in T1DM incidence in females after puberty might be due to increased estrogen activity; indeed, a decrease in estrogen activity is observed in female T1DM patients and at least some of the problems observed in T1DM women may in part be due to the relationship between decreased estrogen levels and insulin action [9]. T1DM onset can be observed at any age [10] but most epidemiological studies focus on the disease with clinical diagnosis during childhood and adolescence. Indeed, adult T1DM may be difficult to discriminate from certain forms of T2DM and from Latent Autoimmune Diabetes in Adults (LADA) [11,12], but in any case the geographical variations of T1DM incidence in adults parallel those reported in children. As we said before, after puberty the incidence of T1DM in women is decreased mainly due to estrogen activity, thus T1DM with adult onset is largely represented in males. In T1DM it is also important to recall that acute diabetes complications like non-ketonic hyperosmolar coma is diagnosed almost twice as often in women compared to men, while hypoglycaemia and diabetic ketoacidosis appears to be 1.5 times more common in females than in males. Rewers and colleagues indicated that the increased risk of diabetic ketoacidosis (DKA) among adolescent girls (relative to younger children) may be related to body image issues leading adolescent girls to skip insulin injections to promote weight loss [13]. Increased insulin resistance due to puberty or obesity may also play a role in the greater risk of DKA, as a higher insulin dose was a predictor of DKA at all ages. Eating disorders, frequent among children with diabetes, may also affect the risk of DKA but may be challenging to identify in this population. In one study using the Diabetes Audit and Research in Tayside Scotland database, it was suggested that poor adherence to insulin treatment in young adults with insulin-dependent diabetes mellitus is the major factor that contributes to long-term poor glycemic control and diabetic ketoacidosis [14]. A particular disease called diabulimia, which consists of the arbitrary reduction or omission of insulin that results in rapid weight loss but puts the patient at risk of ketoacidosis, has been described as being more common among diabetic adolescents in whom prevalence of this disturbance reaches up to 38% in females compared to the estimated male prevalence of 16%.

4. Chronic Macrovascular Complications in Diabetes

Gender differences are particularly expressed also in diabetic chronic complications. Patients with diabetes have higher incidences of MI than those without diabetes [15]. Diabetic women have a higher risk of cardiovascular mortality, especially in the post-menopause stage, and it is clear that diabetic women lose their normal premenopausal protection against cardiovascular disease. Several studies show that the diagnosis of diabetes is made later in women, who, remaining exposed for a longer time to "uncontrolled" diabetes, have worse clinical conditions at diagnosis than men, with more severe obesity and less ease reaching the desired therapeutic targets. Women are also less likely to receive all diagnostic and therapeutic measures than their male counterparts, and mortality and disability after a first cardiovascular event are known to be higher than in men [16], particularly in the age range under 54 years. Interestingly, T2DM men had higher incidence rates of ST-segment elevation myocardial infarction (STEMI) and non-ST-segment elevation myocardial infarction (NSTEMI) than T2DM women as observed also in the general population [17]. Several studies have found an increased risk of death after myocardial infarction (MI) in patients with diabetes compared with those without diabetes, independently from T1DM or T2DM [18]. In two studies a sex-based difference has been found in a STEMI cohort with a 30-day higher mortality among women, whereas in a NSTEMI cohort and an unstable angina cohort mortality was lower among women [19,20]. Contrary to type 2 diabetes, which is usually characterized by increased cardiovascular risk due to overweight/obesity and increasing age, the literature on the potential sex and gender differences in type 1 diabetes concerning cardiovascular risk factors, metabolic control and drug therapy is scarce.

5. Chronic Microvascular Complications in Diabetes

As the role of sex hormones in chronic macrovascular complications is rather clear, the role in the field of microvascular complications is still an area of uncertainness. We do know that diabetic nephropathy progresses at a faster rate in diabetic females compared with diabetic males and women benefit less from treatment than men do. The connection between diabetic nephropathy and cardiovascular disease is in line with the increased cardiovascular disease seen in diabetic women.

In T2DM, sex-gender differences in diabetic retinopathy are still not very clear in the literature. In a recent paper by our group in more than 20,000 Sardinian type 2 diabetic patients, we highlighted how female T2DM, despite having a higher number of risk factors for diabetic retinopathy (elevated glycated haemoglobin, longer diabetes duration, hypertension), has less diabetic retinopathy than the male patients [21]. But this is true for T2DM, while in T1DM data are more scared and it appears that female might have a faster progression, more than difference in prevalence of retinopathy.

6. Pharmacological Treatment in Diabetes

Of note, none of the randomized clinical trials done so far, are primarily designed to assess sex gender-differences in the benefit from a specific intervention strategy, de facto excluding fertile women from experimentation. This is a very import issue since usually drugs are tested mainly in men and women after menopause and the results are applied to fertile women, where they haven't really been tested. Further characterization of these differences in glucose homeostasis, might enable us to understand new factors that could be fundamental, both to prevent diabetes, and to find adequate and precise therapy for diabetes and for the prevention of its complications. Some sex-gender difference in drug use come from the observation of real-world life. Metformin is able to increase plasma lactate levels significantly higher in female than in male patients, thus, women with diabetes should deserve a greater caution than men when treated with metformin, with the aim of preventing lactic acidosis [22]. On the other hand a recently published paper has shown that female patients seem to be more responsive than males to the cardiovascular protection offered by metformin [23], and again metformin seems to have a protective effect from breast cancer in women [24]. Thiazolidinediones therapy raises the risk of bone fractures more frequently in women, while regarding a new class of drugs, namely dipeptidyl-dipeptidase-4 (DPP4) inhibitors a reduction in bone fracture independent from sex-gender has been found [25,26]. Regarding drugs targeting the RAAS [(angiotensin converting enzyme inhibitors (ACEs) and angiotensin receptor blockers (ARBs)], they may prevent cardiovascular events more efficaciously in men than in women, and again women are less responsive to aspirin treatment than men in trials aimed at primary prevention of cardiovascular events [27,28].

Large-scale trials focused on the pharmacological treatment of micro-macrovascular complications are needed to evaluate the differences in treatments according to sex-gender, in order to develop new gender-oriented molecules. To date, we only know that some drugs are less effective or less tolerated in women. The lack of knowledge of the exact initiation mechanism of diabetes is the main cause of the partial failure on microvascular complications control in diabetes and this is also true for gender-oriented medicine.

Epigenetics has amply demonstrated how present and past experience sometimes indelibly marks our body. For a gender-oriented medicine, it is necessary to put together multidisciplinary teams where the most varied skills can be expressed.

Other aspects, such as gender differences according to ethnicity, migration and psychological aspects, are generally little studied. These topics will be addressed in detail by specific papers that will be included in this special issue.

Men and women are different in behaviour, in the expressiveness of emotions and in certain specific cognitive abilities: men are more rational, women are more intuitive. Even with respect to emotional intelligence, men and women do not differ in empathically recognizing the mood of the partner in the couple, but the difference lies in the fact that men are more reluctant to show their emotions, minimizing them. Environmental and cultural conditioning probably favour differences in the expression of emotions, while women feel free to express themselves through body language and facial expressions. These psychological sex gender differences are important in terms of reaction to the disease and compliance to drug treatment.

Adherence to drug treatment implies of course patient and physician collaboration, thus emphasizing the role of patient and care provider dyads. Nevertheless, guidelines do not deeply consider the sex-gender of care providers, forgetting that he/she is a person and every individual is sexed and gendered. However, the importance of the sex-gender of a care provider is emerging [29]. The influence of physician sex gender in health quality is known since a long time. In particular, several years ago in a large survey it has been concluded that women are more likely to undergo screening with Pap smears and mammography if they are under a female rather than a male physician, particularly if the physician is an internist or family practitioner [30]. Physician gender influences quality of care in patients with type 2 diabetes. Female physicians providing an overall better quality of care, especially in prognostically important risk management [31].

7. Conclusions

Greater knowledge and awareness underlying these premises, will allows to orient ourselves towards realization of an optimal path of personalized/precision medicine, which goes beyond just biological data, including the socio-biographical context where the person lives. To move towards gender-oriented medicine, it is necessary to put together multidisciplinary teams where the most varied skills can be expressed. In order to reach equity between men and women, sex-gender epidemiological reports, preclinical and clinical research are mandatory to evaluate the impact of sex-gender on the outcomes and to improve sex-gender awareness and competency in the health care system. It is mandatory that future studies should consider sex-gender differences in the setting of randomized controlled trials with drug.

This is why, during the two days, of the virtual web-meeting GENDER DIFFERENCES IN DIABETES held in Olbia, Italy the 4th and 5th of December 2020 (https://www.simdoeducation.com/on-demanddifferenzedigenere, accessed on 5 December 2020), different specialists, psychologists, psychotherapists, anthropologists, cardiologists, diabetologists, nephrologists, nutritional biologists and pharmacologists with experience in the field, coming from different regions of Italy, have discussed the topic of gender differences, to emphasize that the sex-gender medicine is not the medicine for women, but the medicine for men and women, for boy and girl. Starting from this meeting, a multicentre observational trial on gender differences to some drugs in Real-Life, will start shortly within the scientific society SIMDO (Italian Society Metabolism Diabetes Obesity).

Funding: This research received no external funding.

Institutional Review Board Statement: Not applicable.

Informed Consent Statement: Not applicable.

Data Availability Statement: Not applicable.

Conflicts of Interest: The author declare no conflict of interest.

References

1. Seghieri, G.; Policardo, L.; Anichini, R.; Franconi, F.; Campesi, I.; Cherchi, S.; Tonolo, G. The Effect of Sex and Gender on Diabetic Complications. *Curr. Diabetes Rev.* **2017**, *13*, 148–160. [CrossRef]
2. Franconi, F.; Campesi, I.; Occhioni, S.; Tonolo, G. Sex-gender differences in diabetes vascular complications and treatment. *Endocr. Metab. Immune Disord. Drug Targets* **2012**, *12*, 179–196. [CrossRef] [PubMed]
3. Rogers, R.G.; Everett, B.G.; Onge, J.M.; Krueger, P.M. Social, behavioral, and biological factors, and sex differences in mortality. *Demography* **2010**, *47*, 555–578. [CrossRef]
4. Bock, G.; Dalla Man, C.; Campioni, M.; Chittilapilly, E.; Basu, R.; Toffolo, G.; Cobelli, C.; Rizza, R. Pathogenesis of pre-diabetes: Mechanisms of fasting and postprandial hyperglycemia in people with impaired fasting glucose and/or impaired glucose tolerance. *Diabetes* **2006**, *55*, 3536–3549. [CrossRef] [PubMed]
5. Drivsholm, T.; Ibsen, H.; Schroll, M.; Davidsen, M.; Borch-Johnsen, K. Increasing prevalence of diabetes mellitus and impaired glucose tolerance among 60-year-old Danes. *Diabet. Med.* **2001**, *18*, 126–132. [CrossRef]
6. Saeedi, P.; Petersohn, I.; Salpea, P.; Malanda, B.; Karuranga, S.; Unwin, N.; Colagiuri, S.; Guariguata, L.; Motala, A.A.; Ogurtsova, K.; et al. Global and Regional Diabetes Prevalence Estimates for 2019 and Projections for 2030 and 2045: Results from the International Diabetes Federation Diabetes Atlas, 9th ed. *Diabetes Res. Clin. Pract.* **2019**, *157*, 107843. [CrossRef]
7. Williams, J.W.; Zimmet, P.Z.; Shaw, J.E.; de Courten, M.P.; Cameron, A.J.; Chitson, P.; Tuomilehto, J.; Alberti, K.G. Gender differences in the prevalence of impaired fasting glycaemia and impaired glucose tolerance in Mauritius. Does sex matter? *Diabet. Med.* **2003**, *20*, 915–920. [CrossRef]
8. DECODE Study Group. Age- and sex-specific prevalences of diabetes and impaired glucose regulation in 13 European cohorts. *Diabetes Care* **2003**, *26*, 61–69. [CrossRef] [PubMed]
9. Codner, E. Estrogen and type 1 diabetes mellitus. *Pediatr. Endocrinol. Rev.* **2008**, *6*, 228–234.
10. Patterson, C.; Guariguata, L.; Dahlquist, G.; Soltesz, G.; Ogle, G.; Silink, M. Diabetes in the young—A global view and worldwide estimates of numbers of children with type 1 diabetes. *Diabetes Res. Clin. Pract.* **2013**, *103*, 161–175. [CrossRef]
11. Tuomi, T.; Groop, L.C.; Zimmet, P.Z.; Rowley, M.J.; Knowles, W.; Mackay, I.R. Antibodies to glutamic acid decarboxylase reveal latent autoimmune diabetes mellitus in adults with a non-insulin-dependent onset of disease. *Diabetes* **1993**, *42*, 359–362. [CrossRef]
12. Zimmet, P.Z. Diabetes epidemiology as a tool to trigger diabetes research and care. *Diabetologia* **1999**, *42*, 499–518. [CrossRef] [PubMed]
13. Duca, L.M.; Wang, B.; Rewers, M.; Rewers, A. Diabetic Ketoacidosis at Diagnosis of Type 1 Diabetes Predicts Poor Long-term Glycemic Control. *Diabetes Care* **2017**, *40*, 1249–1255. [CrossRef]
14. Neumark-Sztainer, D.; Patterson, J.; Mellin, A.; Ackard, D.M.; Utter, J.; Story, M.; Sockalosky, J. Weight control practices and disordered eating behaviors among adolescent females and males with type 1 diabetes. *Diabetes Care* **2002**, *25*, 1289–1296. [CrossRef]
15. Millett, E.R.C.; Peters, S.A.E.; Woodward, M. Sex differences in risk factors for myocardial infarction: Cohort study of UK Biobank participants. *BMJ* **2018**, *363*, 427. [CrossRef]

16. Gregg, E.W.; Gu, Q.; Cheng, Y.J.; Narayan, K.M.; Cowie, C.C. Mortality trends in men and women with diabetes, 1971 to 2000. *Ann. Intern. Med.* **2007**, *147*, 149–155. [CrossRef]
17. Walli-Attaei, M.; Joseph, P.; Rosengren, A.; Chow, C.K.; Rangarajan, S.; Lear, S.A. Variations between women and men in risk factors, treatments, cardiovascular disease incidence, and death in 27 high-income, middle-income, and low-income countries (PURE): A prospective cohort study. *Lancet* **2020**, *396*, 97–109. [CrossRef]
18. Schmitt, V.H.; Hobohm, L.; Münzel, T.; Wenzel, P.; Gori, T.; Keller, K. Impact of diabetes mellitus on mortality rates and outcomes in myocardial infarction. *Diabetes Metab.* **2021**, *47*, 101211. [CrossRef] [PubMed]
19. Berger, J.S.; Elliott, L.; Gallup, D.; Roe, M.; Granger, C.B.; Armstrong, P.W.; Simes, R.J.; White, H.D.; Van de Werf, F.; Topol, E.J.; et al. Sex Differences in Mortality Following Acute Coronary Syndromes. *JAMA* **2009**, *302*, 874–882. [CrossRef] [PubMed]
20. Kautzky-Willer, A.; Hintersteiner, J.; Kautzky, A.; Kamyar, M.R.; Saukel, J.; Johnson, J.; Lemmens-Gruber, R. Sex-specific-differences in cardiometabolic risk in type 1 diabetes: A cross-sectional study. *Cardiovasc. Diabetol.* **2013**, *12*, 78. [CrossRef]
21. Cherchi, S.; Gigante, A.; Spanu, M.A.; Contini, P.; Meloni, G.; Fois, M.A.; Pistis, D.; Pilosu, R.M.; Lai, A.; Ruiu, S.; et al. Sex-Gender Differences in Diabetic Retinopathy. *Diabetology* **2020**, *1*, 1–10. [CrossRef]
22. Li, Q.; Liu, F.; Zheng, T.S.; Tang, J.L.; Lu, H.J.; Jia, W.P. SLC22A2 gene 808 G/T variant is related to plasma lactate concentration in Chinese type 2 diabetics treated with metformin. *Acta Pharmacol. Sin.* **2010**, *31*, 184–190. [CrossRef] [PubMed]
23. Lodovici, M.; Bigagli, E.; Luceri, C.; Mannucci, E.; Rotella, C.M.; Raimondi, L. Gender-related drug effect on several markers of oxidation stress in diabetes patients with and without complications. *Eur. J. Pharmacol.* **2015**, *766*, 86–90. [CrossRef] [PubMed]
24. Guppy, A.; Jamal-Hanjani, M.; Pickering, L. Anticancer effects of metformin and its potential use as a therapeutic agent for breast cancer. *Future Oncol.* **2011**, *7*, 727–736. [CrossRef] [PubMed]
25. Kahn, S.E.; Haffner, S.M.; Heise, M.A.; Herman, W.H.; Holman, R.R.; Jones, N.P.; Kravitz, B.G.; Lachin, J.M.; O'Neill, M.C.; Zinman, B.; et al. Glycemic durability of rosiglitazone, metformin, or glyburide monotherapy. *N. Engl. J. Med.* **2006**, *355*, 2427–2443. [CrossRef]
26. Monami, M.; Dicembrini, I.; Antenore, A.; Mannucci, E. Dipeptidyl peptidase-4 inhibitors and bone fractures: A meta-analysis of randomized clinical trials. *Diabetes Care* **2011**, *34*, 2474–2476. [CrossRef]
27. Rabi, D.M.; Khan, N.; Vallee, M.; Hladunewich, M.A.; Tobe, S.W.; Pilote, L. Reporting on sex-based analysis in clinical trials of angiotensin-converting enzyme inhibitor and angiotensin receptor blocker efficacy. *Can. J. Cardiol.* **2008**, *24*, 491–496. [CrossRef]
28. De Berardis, G.; Sacco, M.; Strippoli, G.F.; Pellegrini, F.; Graziano, G.; Tognoni, G.; Nicolucci, A. Aspirin for primary prevention of cardiovascular events in people with diabetes: Meta-analysis of randomised controlled trials. *BMJ* **2009**, *339*, b4531. [CrossRef]
29. Domenighetti, G.; Luraschi, P.; Marazzi, A. Hysterectomy and sex of the gynecologist. *NEJM* **1985**, *313*, 148–153.
30. Lurie, N.; Slater, J.; McGovern, P.; Ekstrum, J.; Quam, L.; Margolis, K. Dose sex of the physician matter? *NEJM 12* **1993**, *329*, 478–482. [CrossRef]
31. Berthold, H.K.; Gouni-Berthold, I.; Bestehorn, K.P.; Bo, M.; Krone, W. Physician gender is associated with the quality of type 2 diabetes care. *J. Intern. Med.* **2008**, *264*, 340–350. [CrossRef] [PubMed]

MDPI
St. Alban-Anlage 66
4052 Basel
Switzerland
Tel. +41 61 683 77 34
Fax +41 61 302 89 18
www.mdpi.com

Diabetology Editorial Office
E-mail: diabetology@mdpi.com
www.mdpi.com/journal/diabetology

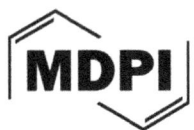

www.ingramcontent.com/pod-product-compliance
Lightning Source LLC
LaVergne TN
LVHW070042120526
838202LV00101B/385